I Swear

www.penguin.co.uk

I Swear

My Life With Tourette's

JOHN DAVIDSON

as told to Abbie Ross

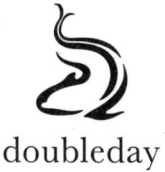

doubleday

TRANSWORLD PUBLISHERS

UK | USA | Canada | Ireland | Australia
India | New Zealand | South Africa

Transworld is part of the Penguin Random House group of companies
whose addresses can be found at global.penguinrandomhouse.com.

Penguin Random House UK, One Embassy Gardens,
8 Viaduct Gardens, London SW11 7BW

penguin.co.uk

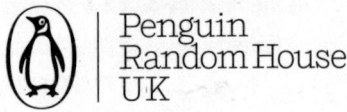

Penguin
Random House
UK

First published in Great Britain in 2025 by Doubleday
an imprint of Transworld Publishers

001

Copyright © John Davidson and Abbie Ross 2025

The moral right of the author has been asserted.

This book is a work of non-fiction based on the life, experiences and recollections
of the author. In some cases names, places, dates, sequences or the detail of
events have been changed to protect the privacy of others. The author has
stated to the publishers that, except in such minor respects not affecting
the substantial accuracy of the work, the contents of this book are true.

Many thanks to Dottie Achenbach and Paul Stevenson for their photographs.
Thanks to Richard Walker of Fabulous Films Limited for *John's Not Mad* DVD
cover artwork. All other photographs are from the author's collection.

Every effort has been made to obtain the necessary permissions with
reference to copyright material, both illustrative and quoted. We apologize
for any omissions in this respect and will be pleased to make the
appropriate acknowledgements in any future edition.

Typeset in 11.1/15.2pt Calluna by Six Red Marbles UK, Thetford, Norfolk
Printed and bound in Great Britain by Clays Ltd, Elcograf S.p.A.

The authorized representative in the EEA is Penguin Random House
Ireland, Morrison Chambers, 32 Nassau Street, Dublin D02 YH68.

A CIP catalogue record for this book is available from the British Library

ISBN: 9781529961850

Penguin Random House is committed to a sustainable future
for our business, our readers and our planet. This book is made
from Forest Stewardship Council® certified paper.

MIX
Paper | Supporting
responsible forestry
FSC® C018179

In memory of Tommy Trotter
1 January 1955 – 3 June 2019

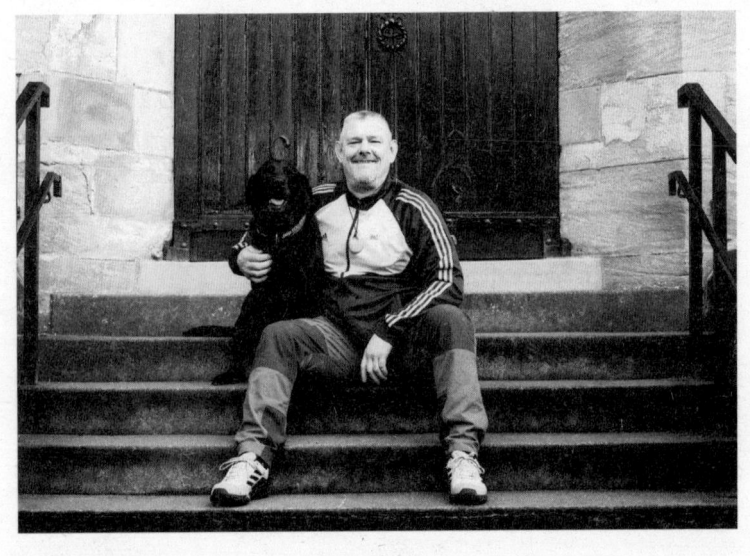

'Hope is optimism with a broken heart.'

—Nick Cave, *Faith, Hope and Carnage* by Nick Cave and
Sean O'Hagan (Canongate Books, 2023)

'In examining disease, we gain wisdom about anatomy and physiology and biology. In examining the person with disease, we gain wisdom about life.'

—Dr Oliver Sacks, *The Man Who Mistook His Wife for a Hat* (Picador, 1985)

'I remember one man with Tourette's, who wrote and said that he had a "tourettised soul", it affects one and one affects it—there's a liaison of a sort. A condition is sometimes a collusion, and sometimes a compromise.'

—Dr Oliver Sacks speaking at the *Music and Brain* presentation
at the 2008 Science Festival, New York City

A Note About Tourette's Syndrome

Tourette's syndrome affects around one in a hundred school-aged children.
It's more common than most people realize – and often goes undiagnosed.
(NHS England, 2023)

Coprolalia – involuntary swearing – affects only around one in ten people with Tourette's.
Though often portrayed in the media, it's not typical of the condition.
(Tourettes Action, UK)

Tics can be motor or vocal, simple or complex.
They range from blinking or throat-clearing to repeating phrases or performing patterned movements.
(NICE Guidelines on Tic Disorders, 2022)

Tourette's rarely appears on its own.
Up to 85 per cent of people with Tourette's also have conditions such as ADHD, OCD, anxiety or autism.
(European Clinical Guidelines for Tourette Syndrome, 2011)

Tics can change over time.
They may increase or decrease in frequency, and often shift in form – especially under stress, excitement or fatigue.
(Great Ormond Street Hospital (GOSH))

People with Tourette's can suppress their tics – but it's exhausting.
Suppressing tics often causes discomfort and can lead to a rebound of more intense tics later.
(Tourettes Action, UK)

Tourette's isn't just a childhood condition.
Although it typically starts between the ages of five and ten, many continue to experience symptoms well into adulthood.
(NHS Inform Scotland)

Repetition is a common feature.
Some people repeat others' words (echolalia), their own words (palilalia), or imitate others' movements (echopraxia).
(DSM-5, American Psychiatric Association)

Tourette's is a spectrum condition.
Some people barely notice their tics, while others experience severe and painful symptoms. Most fall somewhere in between.
(NHS England, 2023)

There is no cure – but there is adaptation, self-awareness and resilience.
Many people with Tourette's report strong creativity, humour and emotional intelligence.
(Dr Tara Murphy, GOSH)

Further Information

NHS England, Tourette's Syndrome Overview, 2023
Tourettes Action (UK), www.tourettes-action.org.uk
NICE Guidelines on Tic Disorders, 2022
Great Ormond Street Hospital (GOSH), Specialist
    Resources on Tourette Syndrome
DSM-5, American Psychiatric Association
European Clinical Guidelines for Tourette Syndrome,
    2011
NHS Inform Scotland
National Institute of Neurological Disorders and Stroke
    (NINDS), 2023

I

The Letter

The letter, when it came, was in a thick, white envelope. It stood out from my usual post – the bills and the junk mail, and the boring stuff like that.

It looked important.

I'm in trouble, I thought. *They've caught up with me now.*

There'd be something I'd done, guaranteed.

There was always something.

The letter was addressed to me, Mr John Craig Davidson, and it said 'Esquire' after my name.

Esquire? Who gets a letter with 'Esquire' after their name? I thought. *What does that mean?*

On the top right of the envelope were the words 'Private and Confidential', and my heart started racing when I saw the Home Office stamp, and 'On Her Majesty's Service' typed in black ink.

This is serious now.

What is it? What the fuck have I done?

I was shaking. My hands were all over the place – that sticks with me, and how tricky it was to open the envelope, like I'd lost control of my fingers.

Suki, my black Labrador, was looking at me, thinking something was up, her tail wagging and thumping on the wooden floor as I ripped it open and made a right mess of it.

At the top of the letter it said 'In strict confidence', and I couldn't help smiling at that, because if you know me, you know there's no way I can keep anything a secret: if I'm not meant to say it, you can bet I'll be straight out with it. Surprise birthday parties are a nightmare for that.

'The Prime Minister has asked me to inform you,' the letter began.

'What's this, Suki?' I asked. 'What does the Prime Minister want with me?'

I always ask her advice, and she's not helped me out yet, but I live in hope.

'. . . Her Majesty the Queen may be graciously pleased to approve that you be appointed a Member of the Order of the British Empire (MBE) in the New Year 2019 Honours List,' I read out loud.

I remember looking around my front room, checking: *Yes, there's my couch with the orange cushions, my mug on the coffee table, the photo of Suki on a canvas on the wall.* Outside: *Yes, the front garden's still there, still real.* A wee robin flitted down on to the bird feeder to prove it.

WHAT THE FUCK?

I just stared at those three capital letters. *MBE.*

Being awarded to me.

Suki was whining now, as I stood there with my mouth open, trying to make sense of it.

Things like this – they don't happen to people like me.

I can slip straight into full-on panic mode if I'm not careful, and so I breathed in deep a few times to calm myself.

Should I be accepting this? I was thinking, as a reel played on a loop in my head: the edited highlights of all those shame-making things from my past that I try hard to keep hidden away.

Is this something I really deserve?

I've worked hard over the years, trying to spread awareness of Tourette's, I've worked really hard, I told myself.

Fuck yeah! I thought. *This is something I'm going to very proudly accept.*

'Guess what, Suki?' She cocked her head at me. 'Daddy's going to go to Edinburgh to accept a medal!' And she jumped up at me, all crazy excited, and started licking my face.

Even on a normal day, it's hard enough for me to keep my emotions in check, but now they were flying all over the place: excitement, then panic, and then that familiar feeling of dread that always overtakes me whenever I have to put myself out there.

It was like I was preparing myself for battle, or embarking on an epic quest. I knew I'd have to dodge so many obstacles first, fighting my way through God knows what chaos of my own making, and then, only then, could I bag the prize.

Dottie, I thought. *I need to phone Dottie.*

Dottie's like my adopted mum, or the godmother I never had. However you want to describe her, she's like family: someone who always has my back.

'Dottie, are you sitting down?' I asked, trying to sound calmer than I felt.

'Aye?' she said. 'Why?' I could tell from her voice she was thinking, *Here we go. What the hell has he done now?*

She just went quiet when I told her.

'Are you still there?' I said, because Dottie doesn't do quiet, not really.

'I'm here, aye.'

'Well, what do you think of that?'

It took me a second to realize that the weird noise she was making, the high-pitched wail, was the sound of her crying.

'Are you OK, Dottie? What's up? Are you all right?'

'Davidson, you daft lad.' She was laughing now. 'Of course I am. I'm beside myself!'

I could invite three people to come with me to the ceremony. For most people, that's probably an easy enough decision – maybe they'd choose their mum, their dad, their partner – but for me, it's never been that straightforward.

I haven't ever had a long-term partner, but that's not through lack of wanting, or trying, but who wants to stay with someone who calls out another woman's name when they're having sex? Or punches them in the breast? Who wants to live with someone who calls out to an obese person in the street with the cruellest taunt they can think of?

Some people think Tourette's is funny, or an excuse to behave badly, but believe me, it's the opposite of how I want to behave. I don't doubt it's impossible to be with someone so eaten up by it, too – all the ups and mainly downs that it creates. So no, sadly, there's no partner.

My parents are still alive, but I don't see too much of them these days. All the years of living with my Tourette's made it hard for them to cope. I get it. I don't know how I would have dealt with me as a son, if I'm honest, so of course it took its toll on our relationship.

When Tourette's arrived, life took on a different shape for us all.

I think back to the meals at the dinner table, me spitting food in my family's faces; the calls from the police; the problems at school; the endless doctors' appointments; the rage from other kids' parents. All that upset and stress and the strain of it. Can you imagine what that does to a family? In the end, my parents' marriage just couldn't survive it.

I still see them both, and I love them, but though things are much better now than they were, we're not close.

Sometimes when I can't get to sleep at night, I can make myself go mad with the guilt of it. I think of what Tourette's did to us all, how it ripped through and destroyed what might have been a happy, functional family. It's hard for me not to take the blame for it. I carry that weight with me always.

Dottie made me read the letter out loud to her twice, and only once I was done did it begin to really sink in.

'Will you and Chris come along with me, Dot?'

I heard the crackling of the cellophane wrapper on her cigarette packet.

'Go on – *will you?*' I said. I have ADHD as well as Tourette's, so maybe it's down to that, or maybe it's just me, but I was born an impatient bastard.

Now I heard the grinding flick of her lighter, and her sharp inhale of a cigarette.

'Dottie!' I said. '*Please!* Will you just answer me!'

'Davidson, keep your hair on, will you, lad? Of course we'll come.' She gave a shriek of laughter. 'We wouldn't miss it for the world.'

'Oh, thank God,' I said, patting Suki's head to calm myself. 'WHORE! Dottie! You're a fucking whore!'

No need to apologize. Not with Dottie. It's such a relief for me to be able to tic shame-free.

Worrying about the third person to take with me was all I could think of for a while. Choosing Dottie and her husband, Chris, had been easy.

They'd taken me in, without question, when I was sixteen and everything had got too much for me. They've played such a massive part in my life, and still do to this day, standing by me and supporting me and giving me so much encouragement and love.

But who else?

There was so much guilt attached to it – all I could think was who I would upset by leaving them out.

Eventually I decided on Caroline, my younger sister, and asked if she could represent my whole family. She's the one I'm closest to out of my three siblings, and the most accepting of my condition.

She was blown away when I asked her, and she started crying too.

I'm going to have to get used to this, I thought, *this happy crying thing. It's all a bit new to me.*

Caroline was in charge of my outfit. Galashiels, where we live in the Scottish Borders, is a big enough town, but it's not big on fancy clothes shops, so we took a trip to Edinburgh, to a specialist place that did all the traditional Scottish clothing.

I was all set on a kilt but, as Caroline pointed out, a true Scot can't wear underwear with a kilt, and knowing I was naked under there would be just too much of a temptation for me. Even the thought of me exposing myself and shouting out 'My crown jewels are bigger than yours!' made me sweat with shame, so I was relieved to settle on a Bonnie Prince Charlie jacket, with a waistcoat and a bow tie, and some lovely tartan trews. They came halfway up my stomach, and I felt a wee bit like Simon Cowell in them, but I didn't care – they seemed like the safest option.

When the day came, Dottie and Chris came with Caroline to pick me up in their blue Volvo estate.

Seeing them all dressed up in their fancy clothes – Caroline and Dottie in their lovely summer frocks, and Chris in his tartan – made my eyes fill up, and I swiped my tears away with the back of my sleeve, embarrassed. I don't cry very much these days. I used to, non-stop, in the early days, but now I think I'm so busy trying to stop things coming out, it's not that easy for me to let go.

When I got in the back seat, the first thing I did was to get the seatbelt on as fast as I could, wrapping my arm in it, trapping it there, just in case I got that compulsion to punch my sister in the face. I gave up sitting in the front seat years ago after grabbing the steering wheel and guiding the car off the motorway at seventy miles an hour.

I remember looking at Caroline's feather headpiece blowing in the wind as we drove off with the windows down, and thinking, *I'm going to bash it*, so I kept the seatbelt tightly round my twitching arm till it went numb and stopped being a bother.

I was fretting in the car for the whole journey to Holyrood Palace, and my ticcing was near constant for a while.

'Wanker!'

'Dottie, show us your titties!'

'Let's have sex!'

'God, John, you aren't half hyper, aren't you?' my sister said. 'It'll be a breeze,' she continued. 'If you panic, just tell yourself, "I've been through so much worse."'

She was right. Compared to some of the things I've had to face, collecting an MBE was like the ultimate quality problem.

The drive to Edinburgh from Galashiels takes you through some grand countryside. We passed mountains and lochs and forests of Scots pines, following the Gala Water for a while, past my favourite fishing spots, where I've lost myself for hours fishing for rainbow trout.

It was blue skies all the way, but the views and the sun warming me through the glass didn't soothe me like they usually would.

Worrying and Tourette's is a dangerous combination. The more you worry about something setting off your tics, the more likely it is that you *should* be worried. It's never a case of 'will I embarrass myself?' It's a case of when, and how badly. When I'm out and about, I'm never more than a split second away from saying something that will get me arrested or punched in the face.

What if the police don't know who I am? I kept thinking. *What if I get chucked out?* Picturing all the disasters I could make happen, the fear of it pushed away any excitement or pride I should have been feeling.

There was a bottle of fizz in the back with the picnic Dottie had packed for the journey home.

'How about we open up that champagne?' I said.

Dottie turned round to smile at me. 'You don't need it. You'll be fine – don't you worry.'

'But I cannae do it.'

'Bullshit, Davidson!' That got me sitting up straight in my seat. 'You'll be amazing,' she said. *'You really deserve this.'*

I remember just staring at the floor of the car.

Edinburgh was so busy that day. I don't do too well with cities as it is: the noise and the crowds and the busyness, all of it sets me on edge.

The traffic was bad. I remember the car slowing to a crawl as we got closer to Arthur's Seat, where the palace is, just below it. I started to get really ticcy as we joined the queue of cars heading to the entrance. There were barriers everywhere, and just the sight of them made my chest tighten; I felt like I was going to burst right out of my waistcoat.

This is it, I thought as we drove through the massive, fancy gates into the grounds. *It's actually going to happen.*

Through the gates, the sandstone walls of the turreted palace threw long, dark shadows across the immaculate lawns. I couldn't believe just how many people there were, all done up in their best clothes, straightening up as they got out of their cars, smoothing themselves down with nervous smiles. Everywhere I looked there were uniformed officials, so smart and serious and professional it was impossible not to feel intimidated.

I hadn't really thought through the sheer scale of the operation.

Armed police were waiting to greet us, and I felt my stomach sinking inside my high-waisted trews at the sight of them.

My tics have got me into so much trouble over the years, so policemen just remind me of what I'm capable of. I've spat at them, punched and sworn at and insulted them, and who was to say I wouldn't do the same today? God forbid I catch sight of a Black police officer . . .

I chewed my lip as I sat there in the back of the car. *Come on now*, I told myself, *keep it together, you can do this* – sitting on my hands, digging my fingers deep into the car seat to stop me from punching the window.

A policeman bent down to Dottie's open window to ask us for our ID, as a couple of other police officers started checking the underside of the car with metal detectors and mirrors, and I felt the panic rising then, and a tic starting to bubble up inside me.

I knew what they were looking for. We all knew what they were looking for. You don't say it, though, do you? You don't alarm people by reminding them of the facts of the matter.

I could see Dottie knew what I was battling with from the way she was staring at me in the mirror, with that steadying, 'easy now' look that she gives me.

I tried so hard to keep the tic back – biting my lip, holding my breath – but sometimes there's no stopping it, and it just blew up and I shouted out:

'Bomb! *I've got a fucking bomb!*'

People stopped what they were doing, and heads turned towards me.

Imagine the shame of saying the very worst thing you can think of.

It makes you want to melt away and disappear into nothing, and sometimes, like in that moment, I can be silenced and frozen by it. It feels like my plug has been pulled out, and I stop functioning.

My expectations when it comes to people's reactions are usually pretty accurate. If they're a stranger, I'm used to their shock and anger; sometimes I get that look of complete revulsion. I think I've had to develop a sixth sense over the years to survive, and I'm proud of that – the way I can read people and be 99 per cent spot on – but I got it wrong when it came to this. The policeman just gave a wry smile.

'Oh, hi there, Mr Davidson,' he said. 'How are you doing?'

There was a collective letting out of breath in the car, and Dottie grinned as she saw the look of relief on my face, and my shoulders drop back down to where they were meant to be.

Maybe he'd seen me on TV, or he'd been given the nod. Either way, who cares – *he wasn't going to arrest me.*

'Right then, Davidson,' Dottie said as we got out of the car. 'Get in there and make us all proud.'

'I'm fucking HERE!' I shouted out, slamming the door of the car. The proud bit might have to wait.

Sometimes it feels like my Tourette's has a character all of its own. Right now, it was like it was testing everyone, checking to see if they knew that I had it.

'I want to go home, Dottie, please let's get out of here,' I said from the side of my mouth.

'John!' she said. 'Stop fretting – look! Everyone knows.'

Another tic came. 'Fuck that!' I yelled out, and then I could see she was right.

People turned to look, but only for a second, and then turned away and carried on like nothing had happened.

That helped to calm me, and I stopped ticing for a while

as we walked towards the huge double doors, where two officials were standing waiting to welcome us.

'Hello. We're delighted you're here, Mr Davidson,' said one, shaking my hand.

'Just take it easy,' said the other. 'Keep calm. You're OK to tic. If you do, I promise you, nobody's going to give you a hard time.'

I wanted to say, *Thank you*. I'd have liked to have said, *You have no idea what that means to me*. But there was an armed policeman, holding his gun, standing right behind them, and I didn't want to risk it, so I just kept my mouth closed tight and gave them what I hoped was a grateful-looking nod as I put a handkerchief over my mouth to help me to control my breathing.

They led us through a massive hallway and guided us along tapestry-lined corridors, to a big, open, lawned courtyard surrounded by pillars. It was filled with the hum of conversation as guests chatted away to each other while they waited in the sunshine.

Maybe it was the pillars, or the archways, but for whatever reason, the acoustics in that space were terrible. I could hear everyone's conversations way too clearly, and I realized then, with a sick-making feeling, that there was also an echo.

The combination of strangers with an echo thrown into the mix felt nightmarish to me.

The embarrassment potential was just too high for me to be able to get any control of my tics.

I remember feeling the pressure building in my stomach and sweat breaking out on my forehead, and having to lean against a pillar to steady myself.

'You're all right, John, you're doing grand.' Dottie put her hand on my arm.

I'm not great with touch, but she knows that sometimes, like right then, I need it.

Trying to suppress a tic is exhausting, and, for the most part, impossible, but still, I gave it a go and started walking around to attempt to distract it.

I could feel the words travelling up my chest. *You can't control me*, I told myself, but my Tourette's ignored me, and now the words were in my throat. *You're not my master*, I thought, but now they were in my mouth, and, timed perfectly, just as there was a pause in conversation, they burst free and I shouted out:

'*I'm a paedo!*'

Usually, I apologize when I tic like that, but 'I'm a paedo!' echoed straight back at me, and my tic jumped in to respond:

'Aye!' I shouted. 'I'm a paedo, too!'

Echolalia is an unwelcome side effect of living with my condition.

'I'm not!' I yelled in reply, as it echoed back to me again.

'I fucking am!' my Tourette's shouted back, as the guests busied themselves in forced conversation to spare me, my cheeks itching as they turned bright red.

Thankfully, I was saved by a chap banging a stick on the ground to get our attention.

'Can all the people who have been nominated for an award follow me, please?' he called out.

Aye, aye, I thought, *get me out of here*, as Dottie and I followed him along another huge corridor with floor-to-ceiling windows with shutters, and tapestry-covered walls.

At the end was a room lined with red velvet chairs and

a white-painted carved wooden ceiling. Huge oil paintings dominated the walls and silver chandeliers hung overhead. I couldn't take my eyes off the patterned curtains – they were so big and heavy – and I wondered about the effort it must take to draw them every day. They could do your back in.

Wherever I looked, there were big, fragile-looking ornaments on plinths, and I went out of my way to avoid them, because you can guarantee my tics will become physical if I'm in punching distance of breakable, priceless antiques.

I was delighted to see that Doddie Weir was there, too – the ex-Scottish rugby union player, who had MND (and has sadly since passed away).

I'd always liked Doddie. He came from near Galashiels, and he'd always stop and say hello to me if he saw me in town. He was such a kind, gentle man, who'd never take the piss out of someone with a disability.

He caught sight of Dottie and me now, across the crowded room, and waved us over.

'Well, how are you doing, Mr Davidson?' he said, putting me at ease straight away, as I introduced him to Dottie, and we blethered on together for ages. He was excited about getting his OBE, he said, too made up about it even to feel nervous about getting up there in front of all those people.

'Nobody's bothering,' he said when I told him how stressed I was feeling, 'so you can call them whatever you want. Anyway, half of them speak with a teaspoon in their mouth so they'll probably no understand you.'

It felt good to be finally able to laugh.

'Come on, let's get ourselves a drink,' he said, nodding to the wine glasses on the table. 'A glass of wine or a wee dram of whisky would be nice, wouldn't it? To help settle the nerves.'

We weren't laughing so hard when we realized that the glasses were only for water. We'd pass on that, we decided – Adam's ale wasn't really going to hit the spot.

The ceremony was due to start, and we were divided into groups of ten and led down another long corridor lined with photographs of past kings and queens. I wanted to slow down and have a good look at them, but there was no time. There was a sense of urgency now, and we had to keep up the pace.

We passed bedrooms with the doors open, and I tried to keep the feeling of overwhelm at bay by imagining the Queen in her curlers and dressing gown and fluffy slippers, chatting to her corgis as she got ready for bed.

When we reached the entrance to the grand hall, an official raised his voice over the orchestra to instruct us not to move until we heard our complete name and the reason for our award being called out by the announcer, and I kept concentrating on my breath, keeping it deep and regular to calm myself.

The music from the orchestra vibrated through my chest as I walked in with Dottie. Everyone else was going it alone, but I got to have her with me as my special companion, and I was so thankful for it.

'Go on, Davidson, you can do this,' she whispered as she was shown to her seat.

I tried my best not to look at the sea of faces as I stood there waiting with my fellow recipients, so I kept my eyes trained on Dottie – and there, just a few feet away from her, stood the Queen.

I knew that she'd be presenting the awards, but I think a part of me just hadn't believed it, because it was still such a shock to see her.

She looked so small – such a tiny figure in this giant, great big room – but she stood out, all the same, in her floral summery frock covered in white and yellow and lime-green flowers.

She looks kind, I told myself as I felt the pressure building. *She looks like my granny*, I thought, taking deep breaths. *Nothing scary about her at all.* But still the pressure kept on building, like a shaken-up bottle of Coke, fizzing away inside me.

I summoned all my powers to try to keep it in, I really did, but it was so, so hard, and then – *whoosh*!

Out it came.

It just exploded out of me, and I shouted out, at the top of my voice:

'FUCK THE QUEEN!'

2

Premier League

I remember when I was a little lad, maybe seven years old, standing with my mum and brother and sisters, watching my dad play football for the local Sunday league team.

I was wearing shorts, wishing I was in trousers, shivering in the cold and the biting wind.

But so what? My knees could freeze to blocks of ice for all I cared, because my dad was playing football, *in front of the whole of Gala* – that's what it felt like – and, right now, he'd been elevated from my usual, everyday dad into a world-famous celebrity.

That's my dad! I kept thinking, looking around to see if everyone knew, my cheeks burning with pride.

He had the ball now and he was dribbling it across the pitch, and people were calling out his name.

'Come on, Dad!' I shouted, louder than anyone, just so they'd know that man with the sideburns and the silky skills was mine.

In real life, back at home, in our semi-detached council house, my dad was a quiet, reserved kind of man. A joiner by trade, I think he was happiest when he was working, more suited to a solitary life than spending too much time with his family. He was shy, really, compared to my mates' dads at least – compared to my mum definitely – but looking at him now, you'd never guess.

He's short, my dad, maybe five foot six, but he looked like a giant to me, so sure of himself and in control, like someone who ruled the world.

YES! He kicked the ball into goal, and everyone went nuts.

That's what I want, I thought, yelling and cheering along with everyone, as I watched the other dads punching the sky and shouting and hugging my dad, slapping him on the back, like he was their hero.

I decided then, with the ease and confidence that comes with youth, that I would definitely, without doubt, become a professional footballer. *And that was that.*

Done deal.

After that, football became everything to me. If my mum couldn't find me, she knew I'd be out in the street, or in our local park, kicking a ball about.

I was part of a group of lads, all united by a shared vision of our future. They all wanted to become professionals too, and were just as sure as me that any time soon they'd be picked from obscurity, and that a life of worldwide adulation was just around the corner. *Easy.* All we had to do was practise.

When we weren't playing football, we were blethering on about all things football, and our undying love for Glasgow Rangers, as we played Subbuteo at someone's house, crowding round the table, joshing and joking and waiting for our turn.

Ossie Ardiles was my hero. I covered my bedroom walls with posters of him, picturing myself playing for Spurs one day too, and the energy fuelled by that hope kept my football obsession alive.

I got good at it. After all that non-stop practice, it would have been weird if I hadn't, I guess.

A couple of young dads started up a team and I got picked, along with most of my mates.

Of course we did. We'd never doubted it.

This was just the beginning.

I remember those times as happy overall. I wanted to be like everyone else, and I *was* like everyone else. I was part of something.

You know that age – it comes to us all – when you start to notice when people are looking at you? It could easily make you painfully self-conscious, but somehow I rode it out. I made sure that I was dressed well, and looking tidy at all times, just the same as everyone. I had the same trainers, all the cool stuff. It was the eighties, so I had the essential parka with the furry hood, and I rode around Gala at top speed on my Skyway BMX. All my mates had BMXs, too.

I was king of the world.

Not that I knew it at the time. I was just me, like everyone else, and there was nothing to sweat about.

If life is good when you're a kid, it isn't something you notice, is it? If it carries along just fine, *it's just life*.

And then, just like that, it wasn't.

3

How It Started

My mum has a theory as to what started it.

I don't know if she's right or not, but I guess I'll keep my mind open to it.

When I was ten, I had to have my tonsils and adenoids out, and, even now, she's convinced it's connected to that.

I'd been having trouble with my breathing for ages, and I kept on getting tonsillitis. Back in the eighties, if you had any bother with your tonsils, they'd whip them straight out at the drop of a hat. That wouldn't happen now, would it? But things were different then – half my class either had no tonsils or a massive beige plaster over one eye . . . what was that all about?

The operation went well, we were told, but once I was discharged, things didn't pan out as expected. I remember sitting in the back of my dad's brown Ford Cortina estate on the journey back from the hospital, relieved at first, so happy to be on my way home, but I began to feel increasingly ill. My body started aching all over and my arms and legs began to feel all floppy and useless, like they were made out of rubber.

Is this normal – to feel so unbelievably heavy? Like the sheer weight of my body is going to make the car seat buckle under me any minute?

By the time we were home I was hot and red and sweating

all over; my temperature was raging. I remember my arms slipping through my dad's hands as he tried to help me out of the car.

Is this what is meant to happen after an operation?

I had no idea. I'd never had one before. No one had had an operation in my family until now, so none of us knew what to expect.

'You'll be fine, son,' my mum said, her frown contradicting her, as my dad sat me down on my bed. 'You just need to rest,' she said, her eyes wide with concern. 'You'll be right as rain by the morning.'

I wasn't, though. The next morning all I wanted to do was curl up in bed and keep warm.

I took paracetamol and rested, and drank all the soup Mum brought me on a tray. I did all the things you're meant to do, but I think all that did was keep the infection at bay, because that low-level flu feeling didn't fully leave me.

Two weeks later I was still not recovered, and was actually feeling worse than ever. My stomach began hurting, more and more, and soon I was vomiting.

I ended up back in hospital, in Edinburgh again, and had to have my second operation in two weeks – this time to take my appendix out.

I recovered quickly from the operation. I was fine physically when I left hospital, and the fever had gone, but the odd feeling didn't go. I began to feel anxious. It wasn't necessarily about anything specific, just a faint, baseline sense of unease, as if life didn't feel so certain, or quite so safe, any more.

Mum is convinced that I must have contracted Streptococcus pneumoniae, and there is a link – albeit a rare one –

between that and appendicitis. She's certain that the infection triggered my Tourette's, and some research does seem to indicate a link there, too.

I don't know what I think. I'm not sure if it would make me feel better, or worse, if I knew that I got it that way. I've become so used to living with the unknown, with never knowing how I'll be day to day – what I might say or do – that I think I've just got used to uncertainty. Maybe that means that I've stopped craving the answers like she does.

4

Abroad

I was still ten when I first went abroad – to the Costa Brava – in the summer before my last year at primary school. My trips in and out of hospital had taken it out of Mum; she needed a proper holiday. We all did, she said. Money was tight, but when Mum wants to make something happen, she just does – she's determined like that. She cut back, putting bits by here and there, so we could have our first family holiday abroad.

It was a big deal at the time – a *massive* deal. I remember going nuts when Mum and Dad told us, running round the kitchen, yelling and whooping, out of my head with excitement, even though I didn't have the first clue where it was. It was *abroad* – that was enough for me – that mythical place I kept hearing about, where it never rained and the sun always shone, and all there was to eat, all day long, was ice cream.

The name Costa Brava sounded super-fancy to me, and I chanted it over and over, until my mum started looking narked with me. 'All right, John, all right!' she said, with a bat of her hand. 'Calm down now, keep your hair on!'

'Where is it, then?' I said, puffed out, sitting down at our Formica table to wipe the sweat off my face.

'It's in Spain!' Sharon, my big sister, was leaning against

the wall with her arms crossed, trying to look cool. She was a teenager now, so wall-leaning and arm-crossing took up a lot of her time. 'Oh my God, John,' she said, giving me her best withering look. 'Don't you know anything? You big wally.'

'Sharon!' Mum said. '*Language!* Please!'

We'd be camping, Mum said, *in a resort*. The word 'resort' set me off again, making me all giddy and filled to the brim with happiness. I couldn't breathe with the thought of it all, and I had to let the pressure out in a long, high-pitched squeak, like a kettle coming to the boil, as my head filled with images of water slides and bright turquoise water and neon-green slush puppies with stripy straws.

Mum said I should go and have a little lie down.

We took the coach to the Costa Brava from Edinburgh. It felt like we were on that bus for ever and ever – on and on it went, for days, it felt like – but nothing could dampen my excitement, which was a shame for the rest of my family, and I guess everyone else on the bus. I found it impossible to sit still and kept getting up and out of my seat all the time. I found it impossible to keep quiet, too.

'Are we nearly there yet?'

'What about now?'

I was driving everyone a bit mad after a while. 'Sit down, John, for goodness' sakes.' Mum just wanted to read her Mills & Boon. 'We've got hours to go yet.'

'Look at them,' she said, nodding towards my brother and sisters, all sitting quietly, good as gold with their puzzle books.

I was always a high-energy kid. If I didn't have a football to kick about, I just never knew what to do with it all, so I'd fidget and chat non-stop. Even then, I guess, I felt a bit different – in that way, at least – from my family.

It's not often, is it, that a place exceeds your imagination? Well, not mine, anyway: an optimistic ten-year-old boy, with a fanciful, vivid inner life which meant I'd often get let down by reality.

Not this time, though.

The resort was beyond anything I'd dreamt up in my head.

My mind just went blank when I first saw it. *What is this place?* I had no frame of reference, nothing to judge it against; everything about it was new to me. It was like being on another planet.

There were fruit trees everywhere – I'd seen apple trees before, but these had peaches hanging off them, and kiwis, and lemons. Tiny lizards darted around my feet. The air smelt different and felt different – it's pretty rare to feel baking hot in Scotland – and even the soil was different: dry and dusty and pale as sand. There were massive spiky yucca plants dotted all over the place, and palm trees – I hadn't been expecting palm trees! – surrounding the biggest outdoor swimming pool I'd ever seen.

I just stood there for ages, finally still, the heat tightening my cheeks, watching all the kids laughing and splashing about in the water.

'Stay away from the edge of that pool now, won't you, son?' Mum said, which only made me want to head straight to it. Even then, I felt drawn to do the opposite of what I was told.

I'll just dip my hand in, test how cold the water is, I told myself, rushing towards the pool, my mum's voice ringing in my ears. I was too filled with excitement – all jittery with it – and I leant way too far forward, too quickly, and fell in, straight away, fully clothed.

That holiday was one of the happiest weeks of my childhood. We all got on. Even Dad looked like he was having a good time. We'd walk to the sea in the day, muck about on the white sand, swim, then go back to the pool, and head to the club-house at night. There were loads of children to play with, too, and I loved being around other kids back then, so I was completely in my element.

I thought nothing of the blinks at first. I remember the first one – a long, hard blink that came from nowhere – just before I was about to dive-bomb into the pool. I didn't give it much thought, and chucked myself into the water. Every now and again another blink would come, but I was busy running around the place. *Maybe it's the sun*, I thought, *my eyes aren't used to it, that's all* – and I asked Mum if I could get some sunglasses.

The sunglasses didn't make any difference, though. The blinks kept coming back. But no one noticed except me, especially now I had the glasses on.

One evening we were all walking back from the beach with our ice creams, when Mum suddenly stopped dead in her tracks, then let out an awful scream.

She'd stepped on a lizard, she said, hopping about, clutching her foot, and it had *bitten her*. I couldn't believe it, but there it was, its mushed-up body in the dust, and there was the blood dripping from Mum's toe. No one – not from Galashiels, at least – expects to be bitten by a lizard, do they? So I don't blame her for going a bit hysterical, and of course Dad was panicking and all over the shop. He was usually so calm in a crisis, but this was totally off his radar – he'd have taken a burst pipe over this any day, I'm sure. He just kept yelling at Mum to *calm down, calm down for God's sake, will you?* He never yelled, and I didn't like what it did to him; he'd gone all sweaty and red in the face. The whole scenario – the blood, the shouting, the state of my dad's face – all of it was just so jarring after the non-stop holiday harmony.

'What a stupid cow!'

It just came straight out of my mouth.

I didn't mean it. I didn't actually think it. It didn't even make sense.

Why did I say that?

My family were all looking at me, open-mouthed, wondering the exact same thing.

'What did you say?' Mum's eyes go really narrow when she's angry, and her eyebrows go sharp and pointy like daggers. She's got the scariest-looking angry face you can imagine.

'Nothing,' I said, too ashamed to look her in the eye, fixing my gaze on the squashed, bloodied lizard instead.

If I'd been looking up, I would have ducked, but now I felt the shock of Mum's hand as she cuffed me hard round my ear, sending my ice cream splatting face down on to the ground.

I was absolutely gutted.

It was a Mr. Whippy with raspberry sauce, and I'd only just started it.

5

Mr Watson

I felt different after the Costa Brava. You know when you come back from holiday, and you look in the bathroom mirror for the first time, and you get that shock, because the last time you were looking in it you were your normal, everyday pale colour, but now it hits you just how brown you've gone? I felt that same thing, but it wasn't just the change in my skin colour that I noticed. I couldn't get enough of my reflection at first – *Look at that tan, mate!* I leant in closer to examine what looked like just the faintest dark shadow above my lip. *Could a moustache be on its way already? To top it all? Could life get any better than this?*

Then I did the blink. It was the first time that I'd actually seen it, and it looked so big, so *weird*, that I recoiled, stumbling backwards away from myself.

'John? Is that you in there?' Sharon was knocking on the door. 'Hurry up, will you? I'm bursting!' She was always wanting to hog the bathroom back then, acting like it was her God-given right.

I blinked again. *I look like a freak!* I wanted to run to my bedroom, shove my head deep under the covers, but I forced myself to stay put. I gave another blink, and then my head jerked and my face went all funny, my mouth stretching wide like a lopsided yawn.

Sharon was banging on the door now, yelling at me, 'What are you *doing* in there?'

'Give me a *minute*, will you?' I needed to keep on looking.

Next time it comes, just stop it, I told myself, gripping the sides of the sink. *Make it go away.*

It was coming again – I could tell this time, I could feel something building. I tried, I ordered myself to stop, but the jerk came back stronger, and now a yelp came with it, too.

Something really bad is happening to me.

I remember exactly how I felt when that thought hit me, how it seemed to drop from my head and through my chest, landing with a sick-making thud in the pit of my stomach.

I'd got a bit homesick now and then in the Costa Brava. It was my first time abroad, so that was bound to happen, I guess, seeing as I'd lived in Galashiels my whole life. I remember what a big, important place Gala seemed to me then, with its tall chimneys and old mills and sturdy sandstone buildings that looked like they'd been there for ever. It's not a massive town, not really, though it's the biggest town in the Borders – *the Gateway to the Borders* – and I think that made it feel like the centre of the world to me. I'd missed the shape of the hills as I walked down the high street, and the clink of the sweet jars in Annie Rudiman's sweetshop; I'd even missed the stink from the old skin works that could turn your stomach if the wind went in the wrong direction.

I loved that summer holiday, but by the end I was even feeling homesick for my wee Victorian primary school. I knew every inch of it, each mark on the parquet flooring, every tree in the playground, all the scribbles dug into the desk lids.

Now I wonder if it was the dependable familiarity of it all that I was yearning for, maybe because there was something starting to change in me.

Back at school, things felt back to normal again for a while. I still had the last of my tan, and I was peeling by now, so everyone wanted to have a good look at me, which gave me a bit of kudos. I remember feeling puffed up at the start of that first term, happy to be in the thick of things again. Me and my gang of mates were all excited to be together, and I slotted straight back in, playing tag and football with them and mucking about. The blinks and jerks were only coming once in a while, and I hid them from sight by just turning the other way.

My behaviour in lessons was harder to hide. Back in class, where concentration was required again after the long, free and easy summer, I became uncomfortably aware of a change in me. I'd started to go a bit haywire. I just couldn't seem to contain myself, that's the only way I can describe it; it was like everything – all my energy, all my thoughts – wanted to spill out of me. I could feel just how much faster my mind was racing. I couldn't hold my thoughts still. I couldn't hold my body still, either. I'd never found focusing easy, but now that everything had ramped up a gear, it felt impossible.

Thank God I had Mr Watson as my teacher that year.

Most teachers would have lost their rag with me. It would have been all too easy – understandable, really – to have taken my behaviour at face value and just seen me as a naughty kid playing up.

But Mr Watson wasn't like most teachers.

He didn't *look* like the other teachers, for starters, in his cosy knitted cardigans and his oversized glasses that he kept having to push back up to the bridge of his nose. Most teachers in our school wore formal-looking office clothes, which to me gave a clear message: *I am the law, fear and revere me*, that kind of thing. Mr Watson didn't need to try that hard. He had a way about him, that quiet confidence, which I responded to. We all did; he had our respect from the start.

He'd notice me struggling to concentrate, sometimes even before I was aware of it.

'John? Can you come and hand the books out?' he'd say, to get me back in the room.

Rather than tell me off, he just found a way to defuse things, with the calm, confident ease of a bomb disposal expert.

He'd see me getting up from my desk, and step in. 'Great, thank you. Yes, John, can you please take these forms to the headmaster's office?' As if we'd already arranged it, and that had been the plan all along.

At home, Mum was flying off the handle a lot, and I hated it. We had a house move coming up – a good one, really – shifting from our wee semi to a new-build council house with a bit more space on a recently finished development. But it had her totally wound up. We'd get shouted at or clipped round the ear for barely anything, and I was stuck in that high-alert feeling the whole time. So being in class with Mr Watson felt like a breather. I always felt a bit steadier when I was around him.

I must have tested him daily, but he never even raised his voice with me. I was keen to please him, which wasn't always possible, but I kept trying as hard as I could, and I think he could see and appreciate that.

He had a way of explaining things that no other teacher had before, or since – which meant that I actually understood – and despite my increasingly scattered mind, miraculously I still managed to do better than I'd ever done at school that year, thanks to him.

Now I think Mr Watson may well have been on the autism spectrum. He was clearly different in some way, and I wonder if he recognized that I was, too? Perhaps he saw a kindred spirit in me. I'll never know. But I think that's how I saw him.

I thought I'd hidden the tics well, but it turns out that Mr Watson had clocked them from the start. He never said anything to me directly, though, sensitively keeping it to himself, until he saw my mum at parents' evening.

'What do you think about these blinks and twitches that John does, Mrs Davidson?'

Mum said she was a bit thrown when he asked her that. She'd noticed them too, she said, but assumed it was just something I did at home, 'playing silly buggers' to wind her up.

'Sorry if he's been acting the clown,' she said. 'I've told him to pack it in, but he doesn't listen; he never has.'

'I'm not sure he can help it,' Mr Watson said. 'Have you ever thought it might be a stress-related thing?'

I don't think that had ever crossed Mum's mind. She was the one who should be stressed, she told him, with all the effort of dealing with me.

'I've noticed that when John gets uptight or excited' – Mr Watson would have been treading carefully, I bet; you have to tread carefully with Mum – 'not only does he struggle with his attention, but the blinking becomes more pronounced. I really don't think he means to do it.'

Later, back at home, filling me in on the evening, Mum told me she was on the fence with Mr Watson's take on it. It was hard to take anyone seriously who wore cardigans like that, she said.

I don't think he means to do it. I couldn't wipe the grin off my face. *Mr Watson gets me.*

He was the best teacher I've ever had. I often think of the kindness and understanding that he showed me. It helped me, not just then, but in the darkest times that followed, when I was desperate, and grasping for those elusive straws. *Anything to make things feel better.* I'd remind myself that someone had understood me once, so maybe someone would get me again, and then, just maybe, everything would be OK. I don't care if it was naive, or stupid even. That tiny boost of hope helped me to keep on pushing through.

What Mum didn't tell me, until years later, was that Mr Watson had told her that he had real concerns about me going to secondary school. He saw there would be issues before any of us were ready to face it.

It must have hit her hard, his comment, because I remember her going to bed dead early after that parents' evening.

'Are you all right in there, Mum? All OK?' I said, hovering outside her bedroom door.

I was sure I could hear her crying.

'Fine, son, absolutely fine,' she said.

And believe me, if Mum said she was fine, that was it – you left it at that.

6

Blinker Boy

Mr Watson was right to be concerned. While my family, and me, all still had our heads shoved firmly in the sand, I think he could tell that it wasn't a passing thing, and of course I couldn't hide it for ever. As soon as the other kids caught on, that would be it: that cat would be out the bag, running riot all over the shop.

I'd become obsessed with keeping it hidden – unrealistic, I know – but I had it in my head that I'd be back to myself before I knew it. *Any day soon, they'll just go*, I'd tell myself, *just you wait.* I'd been doing my best to try to hide it, but there was only so much I could do. I started to distance myself from my mates, bit by bit, just in case. *Until I'm normal again*, I'd tell myself, *then I'll be back with everyone like nothing happened.*

Everyone at primary school was divided into friendship groups. Even the quieter ones had their own gang; no one was left out. As my last year at primary school progressed, I could tell that the hard nuts – the kids you wanted to stay the hell away from – had clocked something was up with me. I could see them sizing me up at playtime, heads cocked, arms crossed.

'Oi! What are you doing that for?' Nathan Johnson, head

of the gang, gave me a hard shove on my back to get my attention.

He had bright red hair, which back then you could get your head kicked in for, but he was hard as nails, and a massive unit, and the son of the principal to boot, so no one would have dared be that stupid.

'I don't know what you're on about,' I said with a shrug, and tried to do another blink, shielding my eyes with my hand this time to make out the sun was blinding me.

It wasn't washing, I could tell. 'Fucking weirdo,' Nathan said, sauntering back to his sniggering lackeys.

That was it. I knew I'd need to be out the gates at the end of the day the second the bell rang.

I'd always walked home with my mates, but lately I'd started walking back on my own, finding different, out-of-the-way routes to avoid as many people as I could. I'd dart out of the school gates ahead of everyone, speeding up if I heard my mates yelling at me to slow down and bloody well wait for them. I couldn't. It was too high risk. I was knackered after the effort of hiding the tics all day, and the more tired I was, the more likely I was to blink, so the harder and more hopeless it was to keep it hidden.

That day I took the long way back, up Mount Street. I remember I was starving, like I often was after school. I was shaking with hunger, and feeling so mad with myself for this stupid situation I was in, having to add on another twenty minutes to my journey when I was absolutely gagging for a Wagon Wheel. They were way bigger back then, properly filling, and all I ever thought about when I got the hunger on.

I was steaming up the road, nearly at the top of it, when I heard a shout from behind me.

'Oi!'

I turned back to see Nathan, and his mate Jordan, running to catch up with me.

The dread that I felt then was the first time I'd felt fear like it. It rooted me to the spot.

I remember telling myself to run, yelling at myself in my head to *go, go, go!* But it didn't make a blind bit of difference.

I knew I was going to get hurt. I could tell from the way he was smiling at me.

'Hey!' he said. 'Wait there, will you?'

He didn't know about my legs not working.

'Do that thing again for us,' he said.

My voice wasn't working either.

'OK, then, please yourself,' he said, and he thumped me hard in the stomach.

The force and the pain of it made me double over, and he waited for me to straighten up before he shoved me against the wall.

The tics overtook me then, and now I had nothing left in me to hide them.

'Blinker Boy!' He was laughing. 'Ha! That's what we're going to call you: fucking Blinker Boy!'

I remember just how chuffed he looked with himself, how he kept looking to his stupid mate for affirmation, who was laughing way too hard, in that phoney way sidekicks do, just desperate to keep on side.

'Look at me, Blinker Boy!'

I did, and he spat in my face.

I wiped it off with my sleeve, and they were both chanting *Blinker Boy* at me now, and taking it in turns to spit on me as I held my hands up, pointlessly, to shield myself.

On the other side of the street, the lace curtains in the front window of a house pulled back, and I caught a glimpse of an elderly woman peering through, frowning with concern. The sight of her jolted me back, and my thoughts reconnected to my body again. *Run, run, run!* My legs responded, finally, as I raced away from them.

I could hear their jeers echoing behind me as I concentrated on the thud of my feet on the tarmac, each one taking me further away from them, tears streaming down my spit-caked cheeks.

One more week, I told myself, running faster than I'd ever done, *one more week of school and then I'm home and dry.* I had sweat pouring off me and I was panting like a dog. *Soon it's the holidays*, I told myself. *I can go and see the doctor and get some medicine.* Just the word 'medicine' soothed me. I was at that age when I still believed doctors could cure anything and medicine was like a magical potion to me. All I'd have to do was take it, then I'd be right as rain and ready for secondary school.

7

Caravan

I was eleven. It was the summer holidays before secondary school and the tics were developing and morphing into something that was impossible to ignore. I was still blinking a bit, but I'd started to jerk, too, and make the odd shout. Nothing, really, compared to what the tics would become, but still enough to mean I'd started to lose my friends.

Now, I wonder if it was them, or if I felt I had to distance myself. I think it came more from me. When you're eleven, it doesn't take much to be mortified, does it? All I wanted to do was to blend in and be just like everyone else – and I was. Me and my mates were cut from the same cloth: same love of football, same kind of house, same clothes, same way of talking. I'd never given it a second thought. That feeling of fitting in just was. I didn't notice it until it wasn't there any more – and suddenly I was on the outside, looking in. I used to be the one in goal, playing every match with my mates. Now I was staying in my ground-floor bedroom, staring out the window, watching them all messing around playing football together on the green without me. I remember a strange new feeling overtaking me as I watched them all laughing and hugging each other, punching the air when the ball went in the net: a twisting kind of ache in my stomach. It took me a while to realize that the feeling was loneliness. I don't think I'd ever felt it until then, not with my big family and my mates, and living in the tight-knit community that we did, with everyone knowing everyone else's business.

Before the tics came, I sometimes used to really want a bit of peace and quiet, just the occasional breather from people in my face all the time, because I'd never had any time on my own.

Turns out it's true when they say that sometimes you have to be careful what you wish for.

They were good lads, my mates, but I could see that I'd started to test their patience, and, God, do I remember just how much I hated that.

I'd always been a loud, outgoing kid, full of energy and inquisitive, wanting to get into everything and test things out. I remember my friend Ryan's dad would give us a lift every week to the Boys' Brigade in his rusty old Austin Allegro. It was a real bone-rattler of a car with a big hole in the floor, and we'd all be crammed in the back – no seatbelts – staring at the road rushing past below us, but it would always be me wanting to shove things down into it, and my mates pulling me back, shouting at me to give it a rest. So I can see why at first my tics looked to them like me just acting up in a bid for attention.

'Why do you keep doing that, John?' Enzo would say when I'd start up with the twitching again. He was the leader of our gang: half Italian, cool and good-looking and the best of us at football, and a nice lad to boot, so we all quietly worshipped him, copying everything he wore and said and did, the way he walked and everything.

'Doing what?' I'd say, trying to play it down, hoping to make him think he'd imagined it, but it never worked.

'That jerky thing you're doing!' He was smiling but looking confused. 'Making your face go all funny and twisted-looking?'

'Oh, *that*. I don't know, it's just something I have to do,' I'd say, trying to make out it was no big deal.

'Well, just stop it, why don't you?' Ryan used to get really wound up by it. 'It makes you look a right bloody spaz!'

Ryan was a thin lad with a ski-jump nose, and the best goalkeeper out of all of us. We never got invited round to his house, because his mum stayed in bed all day, and we just accepted that and never asked why.

Sometimes I'd just laugh it off and play the fool, exaggerating the tics so they'd think I was clowning around, but that just made things worse and kept them believing I had some kind of choice in the matter.

'You're pissing us off now, John.' Eric liked to drop his voice to sound all commanding and important. He was taller than us and had a different accent, because he wasn't from Galashiels like the rest of us – he was from a town a while away, so we all thought he was dead exotic, and I think he played on that. His mum was a nurse and did night shifts, and Eric spent a lot of time out playing on his own while she was sleeping and had to let himself quietly in and out of his house. We knew never to knock on his door. Except sometimes I just couldn't help myself and I'd go banging on it to try to fetch him, and that used to piss him off a bit, too.

I felt like I was increasingly being seen as a pain in the neck by everyone, which was ironic, really, as I was getting actual near-constant pain in my neck from all the twitching.

My family had been living in our new home in Kilnknowe Place for about six months by then. We called it the upside-down house, because everything was the wrong way round: the bedrooms downstairs and the kitchen and sitting room upstairs, which seemed off-the-scale fancy to me. I couldn't believe it when I first saw it. I thought we'd arrived. I think we all did. It just felt so modern and out there, compared to the house we'd moved from. My mum spent a lot of time making it look nice. How things look has always been impor-tant to her, and she was constantly doing it up – wallpapering, painting, landscaping the garden – on a never-ending quest to make it look perfect. And it did.

My mates were all dead impressed by my house, too, which made me proud, so when we were first in, I was always sug-gesting they come to mine to play. Since the tics had started to get bigger, though, I'd stopped asking them over. It just didn't feel comfortable any more. At least if I was round at someone else's, I could always run back home if it got too much.

At the start of the summer holidays after primary school, we started hanging out a lot at Callum's house instead. He was a quiet lad, who, when I look back now, might well have been on the autism spectrum. He suffered quite badly from eczema, and I remember he was always covered all over in cream. His mum was a nurse, too, and she did night shifts, so we were told we had to keep quiet when we went round there, or we'd be thrown out. As my tics progressed, the thought of needing to be quiet got me more and more het up, but I didn't want to miss out.

We'd all be squeezed in around Callum's Subbuteo table, getting into the game, and then: '*HEY!*'

I'd always yell out at the wrong time, when there was no goal or anything. I wasn't trying to put anyone off their game, but it definitely looked that way.

'*JOHN!*'

I got so used to hearing my name being shouted out like that: full of frustration and despair.

'*SHUT IT, WILL YOU?* Callum's mum's sleeping, remember? We'll all get chucked out!'

'Sorry, lads,' I'd say, shaking my head, looking at the floor – *the shame of it!* 'Sorry. I didn't mean to.'

Sorry, sorry, sorry. That was all I'd say back then, every sentence littered with my abject apologies. Can you wear a word out? How many times can you keep saying the same thing and expect anyone to believe you, when you do the exact same thing a few minutes later?

Soon I was turning down the Subbuteo invites, always giving some excuse. I had a sore belly, or a headache – *thanks for asking, though. Maybe next time.*

Mum and Dad started noticing I was home a lot more.

We'd started going to the doctor's regularly now, Mum and me. The first time I was apprehensive – I'd never liked going to the doctor's – but excited, too, convinced there'd have to be a quick fix for me. But the GP dismissed us from the outset. *It's just a habit*, he said. *He'll grow out of it. It's nothing to worry about. Lots of children have habits like this. And the blinking? Just get his eyes tested; I'm sure you'll find he needs to wear glasses.* Mum would try to argue her point, but was met each time with the same response: *Just be patient, don't worry, it'll go soon.* Each time we'd leave the surgery, I'd be trying not to cry, and Mum would be doing her best to hold it together, too, but I'd notice she'd march out a little quicker, her jaw always set tight with frustration.

'What are you doing inside again?' Mum would shout down the stairs when I'd shut myself in my bedroom, curtains closed. 'Go on, John, get out and play, will you?'

'*I don't want to!*' I'd shout through my door, thinking, *Don't come in, please! Just leave me be.*

'Johnnnn!' Mum had started to say my name like this: all loud and elongated, like it had an exclamation mark after it.

I could hear the drumming of her feet on the stairs, louder and louder, and now she was in my room, frowning down at me as I lay on my bed. Her face always looked like this these days: two permanent big deep creases between her eyebrows, purple shadows under her eyes.

'You can't shut yourself away all the time like this, John!' I hated it when her voice went like this, all squeaky high and whispery and desperate-sounding. 'You've got to get out of the house now! You'll be starting Gala Academy soon,' she said, yanking back the curtains, making me wince and hide my face in my duvet as the sunlight flooded in. 'Before you know it, you'll have to be up and out the door every day, son!'

Mum was usually distracted when she came into my room – *our* room; I shared it with my younger brother, William – her words trailing off as she gathered up the half-drunk cups of tea by our beds, tutting and scolding about the mess as she stacked up our left-behind water glasses. Now, though, she just focused on me, her fists bunched up tight and shoved deep in the pockets of her pale yellow housecoat.

Serious.

'Why don't you want to be out and playing, son?'

'I don't know,' I answered honestly.

'Look at it! It's a lovely day out there. Everyone – Callum, Enzo – they're all out there playing football.'

My face was contorted by blinks and twitches.

'It's time you stopped with this nonsense, John,' she said. 'You do know that if the wind changes, you'll stay like that, don't you?'

That was a terrifying thought to me – being stuck for ever with a frozen, gurning face – and the terror that I felt made me blink and twitch harder and faster than ever.

I didn't know what was happening to me.

I didn't know why I was ticcing.

I didn't know why I didn't want to go out.

I felt like I didn't know anything any more.

That summer was also when the compulsions kicked in.

I started going to walk the dogs in Victoria Park, where the playing fields were, mainly to get my mum off my back, but I felt calmer when I was out of the house and on my own, which was a new and unexpected thing for a kid who'd loved to be in the thick of it. We had two dogs then – Bonny, a Boxer-Labrador cross, and Honey, a black-and-tan puppy, who was also a cross: part Labrador, part God knows what, but she was gorgeous whatever she was. I really loved those dogs. I think I found it soothing to be in charge of something, when the rest of my life felt increasingly out of my control. When I was walking the dogs, I needed to look after them and make sure they were OK. I liked that responsibility. *They* trusted me, at least.

But then Mum would want to come along with me, which made it a lot less relaxing. One day, when I was walking with her, a new tic arrived.

I found myself yanking the dogs' leads, again and again.

'Stop it, John! What are you doing?' Mum had a habit now of pressing her fingers on her temples when I was 'driving her to distraction', as she'd say. I didn't like her doing it, because crying would usually come next, and I didn't want her crying at me again – not outside, where people might see. I couldn't stand the thought of that. A crying mum. How embarrassing would that be?

But still I had to keep on yanking, Bonny and Honey rasping as their collars pulled tight on their necks. *I'm hurting them! What's happening? Why can't I stop?* I was so knackered, so worn down by this confusing disconnect between the thoughts that whirled around inside me and their powerlessness to stop my actions.

'Give me those leads,' Mum snapped as she grabbed them from me.

And that was all it took: the one soothing pursuit I had was over.

Maybe it was a response to that – the overwhelming fear of having nothing left now to help me – but from nowhere I had a sudden strong desire to skip.

The thought of skipping filled me with horror, but the horror of that thought just made the feeling stronger.

I just have to. Don't do it! But I need to! Rational and compulsive thoughts jostled for attention. *Just do it!* And that was it: I was skipping down the road now, hating myself, my mind still battling but failing to control my body that was betraying me.

'John! For God's sakes, *what are you doing?*' my mum hissed from behind me.

Believe me, public skipping when you were an eleven-year-old boy in Galashiels in the eighties was about as high risk an activity as you could get. I think even any one of my mates – and they were good lads, all of them – might have given me a good slap if they'd seen me.

A group of lads, all older than me, were coming towards us now, shoving each other and laughing, taking long hard drags on their fags.

'Stop it, will you, John? People will see!' Mum yanked me by the arm to a standstill. Too late.

'Fucking pansy,' one of the lads muttered as they passed us.

I had to look the other way to hide the tears spilling out from my eyes, rolling down my cheeks – *like a baby! Like a stupid little baby. Not a cool, eleven-year-old lad like me. Come on, John, sort yourself out*, I told myself.

We walked in silence after that, Mum with the dogs, with her 'do not disturb' look on: frowning, mouth set tight and straight so her lips disappeared. *No worries, I'll stay well clear*, I thought, hanging back a little behind her so I didn't feel obliged to fill the silence.

I didn't want to talk to her anyway.

There was nothing to say. There was no explanation to give.

We stopped for the dogs to sniff around a lamppost. *Touch it*, I said to myself, *touch it, to make this feeling go away*, because since those lads, since that humiliation and my mum's upset, a pressure had been developing inside me, a tension, like a sneeze building. The dogs were wagging their tails excitedly, as if the smell of other dogs' urine was the biggest treat ever, which, I guess, to them it actually was.

Touch it! My arm shot out, and with the split-second shock of the cold grey metal on my fingertips, relief flooded through me.

Find the next one, I thought, picking up my pace, skipping again. *What the hell?* One skip, two. *Find the next one*, I thought, *touch it again. Yes*, I thought, *yes! That's what I need to do.*

A couple of weeks into the holidays we were heading back to my grandparents' caravan in Skegness – same as most summers, apart from the previous year when we'd gone abroad. This time it was just me and my mum and my brother and sisters, and Dad would be staying at home. We weren't told why, and we didn't ask. I guessed it was because Mum and Dad had been rowing a lot more lately – mainly about how to deal with me, from what I could make out – and Dad kept on leaving us to it, heading off to the pub all the time. Maybe a little break from me would be good for him, and good for Mum and Dad too, I kept thinking.

The caravan was on a lovely site, right in the middle of beautiful, wild countryside. We were all dead excited in the car, chatting away about what we'd get up to when we got there: which tree to climb first, or should we muck about in the stream? Maybe build a fire? When we'd been there the summer before last, we'd loved every minute of it.

I didn't feel like I'd expected as we pulled up outside the caravan. I waited for it to come, but the thrill just wasn't there. Instead, I felt my stomach sink with disappointment as I watched my mum unlock the caravan's door, and I had a creeping sense of unease as I followed her up the steps. There was nothing different about the caravan; it was the same familiar space, everything as immaculate and unchanged as ever, every trinket just where it was meant to be. Nothing had altered, I realized, but me.

'I want to go home,' I told myself, under my breath.

Last time it had been a right laugh being crammed in all together, but now as my siblings shoved past me, battling to bagsy the top bunks, the thought of being so close to everyone filled me with panic.

Me and my brother, William, ended up with the bottom bunks, of course, and my sisters got the top bunks, like they always did, while Mum had the big bed in the dining area. As we all jostled around in the tight space, shoving our bags on beds, I didn't like the feeling it was bringing out in me: a tic-inducing tension that made me sweat all over with the effort of trying to dampen it down.

We'd arrived late, so soon we were tucked up in our tiny, hard beds.

As soon as Mum put the lights out, all I could hear was my breath. The darkness seemed to amplify it – it sounded so much louder than everyone else's, and I started to become hyper-aware of it. I could feel myself blinking and the twitches starting up again.

I could tell everyone was dropping off to sleep. *I mustn't shout out*, I kept thinking, *I have to keep quiet.* If I woke everyone, there'd be trouble, and not just from William – who was well and truly over sharing a room with me by now – but *everyone* would be down on me like a massive ton of bricks.

The more I thought about it, the more anxious I felt, and

the anxiety and fear of breaking that silence became unbearable, and there it was again: the pressure in me, building and building.

'CUNT!'

I slapped my hand over my mouth in horror. *Oh good God, no! Where did that come from?*

'No!' Mum sat bolt upright, then switched on the light.

'John Davidson, how dare you?' she said. 'We. Do. Not. Swear. In. This. Family!' It was the way that she said it, so slowly, and in a whisper – no shouting – that made all the saliva dry up in my mouth.

She was right. We didn't. Swearing was the worst thing you could do in our family. And that was the worst word. *I mustn't say the worst thing!*

'*CUNT, CUNT, CUNT!*'

I don't think I'd ever seen Mum look that angry. It wasn't just the harsh caravan lighting, either; her cheeks had gone dead pale, all the blood drained from her face. She was white with rage.

'You should be ASHAMED of yourself, John. That's disgusting!' Her voice echoed and bounced off the tin walls.

Everyone was awake now – my brother, my sisters, all wincing in the light, staring at me with confused irritation. That just made me have to keep on going.

'CUNT, CUNT, CUNT!'

'Why are you doing this to me, John?' Mum looked so desperate with her head in her hands. I couldn't stand it.

I was going to ruin her holiday. *I can't ruin my mum's holiday.* I knew how tired she was – I was all too aware of that – how hard she worked, all the cooking and the cleaning, and with Dad buggering off to the pub at the drop of a hat. I could see how much that took out of her, and that was even before I'd started going wrong. I didn't want to be the cherry on her cake, the straw on her camel – or whatever, you know what I mean. She was a sturdy, strong-looking woman, my mum, but physical strength makes no odds in a situation like this. I was fretting that her mind might just break with the stress of it all.

This was how things went when it came to Mum. I'd flip from fear to love and back again. A few seconds earlier she'd scared the hell out of me, but now I just wanted to hug her tight and never let her go.

I cried myself to sleep that night, as quietly as I could, hoping no one would hear me. They must have. You could hear every sigh, snort and cough in that tiny little space, but still, no one said a thing to me. They were all sick of me, I don't doubt, and grateful, probably, that I was at least trying not to disturb them.

I was the first one up the next morning. I couldn't wait to get outside. Briefly, as the crisp air hit my cheeks, it all felt good again, like it was meant to. The sun was out, and ahead of me the view stretched for miles. *All that newness!* The jagged lines of pine trees, and fields that went on and on. *So much green – how much green can you get?* I waited to call my brother and sisters, taking in the quiet for a moment, the unbelievable peace of the place. No traffic, no people, just the odd squawk of a distant pheasant.

Finally, I felt that 'I'm on holiday' feeling. 'Come on, you all!' I yelled up the caravan steps. 'Get up, let's go play!'

Hide-and-seek was always our favourite game when we were there. The place was made for it, with all those trees and bushes to hide behind.

This time, when it was my turn to hide and I was crouched behind a pine tree, my heart beating in my chest with excitement, I tried to keep as quiet as I could, but it didn't work. *I didn't work.* I started ticcing, letting out grunts and yelps.

'John! You idiot!' William was standing over me in seconds, shaking his head in disbelief. 'What did you do that for?'

I used to be so good at keeping quiet. I'd been the undisputed king at hide-and-seek.

I left them to it after that and headed off to the woods on my own, and sat there on a log till the dusk came.

I couldn't wait to get back home. I was wishing the days away for the rest of that holiday, counting the time until I'd be back in my bedroom, picturing the space of it – how far away William's bed was from me, how relaxed I'd feel as soon as I got there.

I didn't, though. I felt all out of sorts when we got home.

The anxious feeling hadn't gone away.

That first night back, I went to bed early – before William, even – just for some peace, and some space, finally, away from everyone. I lay there, exhausted, staring up at my ceiling, which was covered in those luminous star stickers that all the kids had in their bedrooms back then. It was still too light outside for them to have started glowing yet.

It's come to this, I was thinking, *I'm going to have to take myself away like this, go to bed early, just to try to keep normal*, as I listened to my family all chatting away together upstairs over the background hum of the television.

I can hear them, I was thinking, *so if I say something, then they can hear me. I mustn't tic. I need to stop myself thinking about ticcing.*

Then a new and troubling thought came to me:

What would be the worst thing that I could say right now?

Good question, my mind replied, rising to the challenge immediately, offering me up three words in an instant, which combined to form a short and deadly sentence, the equivalent to a hand grenade if they were to be let loose from my mouth in that house.

I tried my best. I bit my lip and pushed my fist tight against my mouth to keep them from bursting out. I swallowed hard to make them go back down, but the power built, like it always did, and the need to release won out.

I shouted at the top of my voice:

'SUCK MY COCK!'

The words echoed round my room.

Upstairs, the chatting stopped.

Now Mum was thundering towards me, and this time there was no reasoning with me, no questions, just a fast, hard slap across my face.

I remember the sound of it reverberating, and the sharp sting of my cheek, then she was gone before I could murmur my pointless apology, slamming my door behind her.

I lay with one hand on my cheek, listening to Mum and Dad upstairs having a one-sided row.

'You've got to discipline that boy!' Mum shouted. 'Come on! Don't leave this all to me!'

Dad mumbled something indecipherable in reply, and Mum was crying now, probably because she knew, just as well as I did, *just as well as we all did*, that she was on a hiding to nothing with that one, because Dad was never one for conflict, never had been and never will be.

It made the way they were together a bit lopsided, with

Mum taking on all the yelling and the slapping for both of them.

Dad had never raised his voice or laid a hand on me before my tics started, and he wasn't about to start now. He just wasn't cut out that way. He's a quiet man, and his response to all this was in keeping with that: he just got quieter and more withdrawn, from me, from Mum, from all of us, really.

He was a hands-on kind of guy – being a joiner suited him – and I reckon dealing with things in a practical way was the only one he knew – his way of keeping his feelings out of it. So he just got up earlier than ever after that, making his sandwiches before any of us were up, then he'd head off out the door so he wouldn't have to talk to us. He'd be back for his tea and, soon after that, straight to the pub, sometimes before he'd even finished what was on his plate if my ticcing was especially bad.

I loved my dad and still do, but part of me used to hate him for withdrawing like that. It's not that I'd have welcomed a double assault – I didn't want him to give me a whack too, or to yell at me, for that matter, either. But it scared me: Mum having to deal with this – and by 'this', I mean me – all by herself.

I used to wonder, if Dad had been more on side with her, maybe she wouldn't have been so frantic and hysterical, and sometimes so out of control with it all. Maybe she could have coped with it better, if both of them had been on board.

It used to frighten me when she got like that, but I get it. There's a limit, isn't there? With all of us. There's only so much one person can take.

8

Fishing

The summer holidays had always flown past, way too fast for me, but I remember that summer just dragging on and on. How to occupy myself had never been something I'd had to think about, but now I just didn't know what to do, and Mum didn't know what to do with me either.

I think it was Mum's idea, to try me with fishing. She must have been desperate – *anything to get him out of the house*, I bet she was thinking. But she knew I loved being outside, and I was always fascinated by how things worked, forever pulling clocks apart on the kitchen table, driving her up the wall. So she went all in and got me a rod and a reel.

I was hooked the second I saw it. I remember feeling properly lit up when she handed it over, like I'd been plugged back in again.

After weeks of not giving a damn about anything, now I was itching to have a go at something – just for a bit, while football was on the back burner, and bikes, and anything to do with my friends, while all that was on hold. Just till I got better from this thing.

*

I taught myself how to do it at first by watching fishermen on TV, taking in every detail, committing it to memory, before going to try it out in real life.

There was a lovely stretch of river nearby, and I headed there as often as I could. I'd find a quiet place, where there were no other fishermen and no one watching me. I was so sick of the feeling of being watched by then.

It was a strange feeling, to still be seeking out solace, and to need it more than ever now, when I'd only ever wanted to be where the action was, when I'd been the most sociable lad of all.

I found a way to go from an outwardly loud, chatty boy to being quietly in my head. It wasn't something I'd chosen, but it's a good skill to learn no matter what, isn't it? To be able to be with yourself, and content in your own company. I'm grateful that I learnt how to do it that summer, and even now, when I need to switch off from the white noise for a bit, I still head there, rod in hand, and can lose myself happily for hours.

Fishing taught me patience. You must think carefully and slowly to be any good at it, and I really wanted and needed to be good at it, so I learnt how to slow my thoughts down.

Later, the more I read up on Tourette's, the clearer it was that I had ADHD too – an all-too-common part of the package – which explained my constantly racing mind. For so long I'd been used to my thoughts going at a hundred miles an hour, but at the riverbank, with no distractions, apart from the odd bright blue dragonfly whirring past, or the flash of a yellow-legged moorhen launching quietly into the water, I felt calm for the first time that I could remember.

The tics would build and multiply when anyone was watching, but I noticed that they came less often when I was alone and relaxed. I found it calming to focus on sounds that for once were nothing to do with me. After a while, my yelps and shouts would die away, and would be replaced instead with other, more welcome noises: the cheery, upbeat song of robins and blackbirds, and the soothing sound of water rushing over the rocks.

Over time I'd try out different things, and I got more skilled at catching fish. I'd work out the most likely places a fish would be in the river, sussing out that where there's a pool, there's usually a big rock, and behind that rock there's likely to be an eddy, where the water's not too fast-flowing, which is exactly where a fish would go to take a break. *I get you, fish, I get you*, I'd be thinking as I cast my rod again, because I needed a break, too, some time out from this overwhelmingly stressful new life that I found myself in.

9

New Start

You would think that a sense of optimism would be helpful in life. But sometimes there is a fine line between being an impressively positive person and a stupidly naive idiot.

Secondary school's going to be a new start for me, I kept on telling myself. *It'll be good for me, I know it will*, I'd think, scrunching my eyes shut, imagining I was casting a spell on myself. If I thought this enough, then you never know, it might just actually happen.

Mum was on about it all the time as well.

'This will be just what you need, John,' she'd say, sounding all flat, like her voice was computerized; doing her best, I bet, to convince herself too.

I can see why we did it. In the absence of any improvement in this mysterious, all-consuming condition that had overtaken me – all of our lives, really – and with signs of it actually worsening, and nothing, no help, from the doctors, we were just desperate, clutching at the spindliest of straws, fixating on the *brand-new-start cure*, which was going to wipe my slate clean and revert me, surely, to my previous, way better, non-malfunctioning self. It just had to happen, because otherwise . . . *what*? I couldn't live with a 'what'. No way. *I'll be fixed soon*. This was the only way I could keep on going.

'Dad and I were saying it's going to suit you much better at the Academy.' Mum was sizing me up in the outfitters' while I tried on the way-too-big school uniform. 'There'll be lots of new people to meet; none of them know anything about you. You can start all over again, can't you, John?'

Now it was starting to feel like a threat: *Don't let me down now, don't ruin this for us, will you?*

'Perfect,' she said, nodding approvingly at my reflection in the mirror. 'You need that bit of growing room.'

'Are you serious? It's, like, ten sizes too big, Mum, please!' I said, waving my arms about. 'Look at the sleeves – you can't even see my hands!'

She bought it anyway.

'I think going to Gala Academy might make me go back to normal. What do you reckon, William?' I was still sharing a room with my younger brother, and even though I was really getting on his nerves these days, it was easy for me to forget – especially when I was tired – and think he still liked me.

'Shut up, will you?' William gave a growl of frustration into his pillow. 'For God's sake, can't you see? I'm trying to *sleep*.' William was eighteen months younger than me, and a quiet, quite shy boy by nature, but I was driving him to distraction by now, and he was pretty much done with me.

'I was just *saying*,' I said, 'I'm looking forward to starting at the Academy, that's all.'

'I don't care,' he said, tugging at his ginger hair in frustration. 'If you don't shut your face, I'll call Mum.'

William and I had a shared sense of humour so we used to have a laugh sharing a bedroom together, blethering away about anything – football, mainly – long after lights out, but I'd been keeping him awake for months with my tossing and turning, and the barks and shouts and funny noises, so whatever I said to him once we were in bed – tic or no tic – was now angrily shut down.

In the days leading up to the start of term, I kept imagining myself walking into the Academy on that first day, head high, smiling at everyone, *back to being me, back to normal*, whatever normal was. It was getting harder for me to remember, the further I got from how I used to be.

What was it like not to be filled with tension and stress every time I left the house?

How did it used to feel? Not to be waiting for the next thing to come out of my mouth?

The memories were slipping away from me, and I kept grasping for them, trying to remind myself, panicking that if I forgot entirely, then my mind would never know how to get me back there.

Most of that first day of secondary school has been erased from my mind. Shock can do that to you, can't it?

'Well? How was it, then?' Mum said when I was back home on the sofa, rubbing the blisters on my heels from my new shoes.

'Yeah,' was all I could give her, because I genuinely couldn't remember. *Thank God*, because the overall feeling was still with me, and it was so unbelievably heavy that all I wanted to do was to drag myself to my bed and go to sleep.

'Do you think you're going to like it?' Her voice was all high and insistent.

'Yeah?' I said, heading downstairs to my room, trying to get away from her as fast as my leaden limbs would let me. I hated lying to my mum, but right now there was no other option.

The day had been everything, all at once. *Now I need nothing, nothing, nothing*, I told myself, tipping face down into my bed.

It hadn't gone anything like I'd hoped it would. Of course it hadn't. I remember lying there, breathing into my mattress and just feeling so *ashamed. What did I expect? How could I have been so stupid?* The jarring difference between my optimistic imaginings and the cold, harsh reality made it all the more painful, and just so very humiliating for me.

It had all been so much worse, in every possible way, than I'd pictured it. Snatches of it came back to me as I lay there, but the memories had a strange, second-hand quality to them, like I was looking in on someone else's life. *This is my life, though.* The tears were flowing and I cried silently, muffling my sobs in my pillow. *This is my life now.*

It hadn't started well, and it just carried on in a steep downward trajectory. I'd been expecting to be put in the same class as my old gang from primary school, but it hadn't happened. Even though I no longer hung out with my group so much – i.e. never – I knew I could still rely on them to be at the very least benign towards me, sometimes even nice. They'd walked into school with me and hadn't laughed at me or completely blanked me, and I was grateful for that. That was as good as I could expect these days.

I remember the panic rising as I scanned the classroom and was met by a sea of strangers, all these new people for me to surprise and shock for the first time. The thought of that made me spasm with jerks. I tried as best I could to hide them, but no one could miss me when I started barking.

'Can you be quiet, please?' The registration teacher was giving me that look – I knew it well by now – of stunned disbelief mixed with fury.

'Didn't my mum say, miss? She said she'd spoken to the school?' I hated the way my voice came out, all reedy high and pathetic-sounding. Everyone, the whole class, was looking at me. 'I have this thing, I can't help it.' I couldn't stand that this was my classmates' first introduction to me. *I'm not just this!*

'Ah, yes, we've been told about you.' The teacher had turned her back on me and was writing her name on the board. 'It's John Davidson, isn't it? Your mother has let us know about your *little habits'* – she spoke really slowly, like I might have trouble understanding her – 'but right now I'm asking you to be quiet and behave, please, while I take the register.'

She doesn't get it. She's never going to get it, either. Tears pricked my eyes, and I had to keep pinching the inside of my hand to tell myself to keep them in.

Crying on day one would be social suicide – on any day, when you're in S1. Reputation-wise, nothing would be worse for me than that.

It was impossible for me to concentrate in lessons, even harder than in primary school. I was so preoccupied with trying to suppress my tics – which, on reflection, given all the effort and stress and tension required, really wasn't worth doing just to reduce or occasionally stop the odd shout or jerk. It never worked enough to stop me attracting attention.

When breaktime came around, I felt like a little animal being let out into the lions' den. I don't think I've ever felt as vulnerable and scared as when I walked out into the playground for the first time.

Just front it out, I told myself. I knew I needed to look the opposite if I wanted to impress potential new friends. *Thick skin, thick skin.* I kept parroting my mum's advice – all I needed to do was grow one, she said, then I'd be fine, then I could deal with anything.

I found a place to stand on the edge of the playground, as close as I could to the door – that way I could run back inside if I needed to – but within seconds I was surrounded by a crowd of kids.

'*Do it, do it!*' A boy from my class began the chant, and now the others joined in. I wanted to put my hands on my ears, but I didn't want to look like it was getting to me, so I let the noise ring in my head as I frantically looked for a way out. There wasn't one.

I'm trapped. As soon as I thought this, the panic made me jerk and I shouted out:

'Cunts!'

The kids started cheering and whooping.

'Fuck!' I shouted. Now the whole crowd was laughing.

'I know what we can call you,' the boy from my class said. 'Cunt Fuck John!'

Some of the kids were screaming with laughter now, doubled up; relieved, most likely, that it was me being singled out, and not them.

'Cunt Fuck John!' they called out after me as I made a break for it, shoving my way through the tangle of arms, head down as I scarpered back inside.

I didn't know where I was going, just away from them all. *I've never run this fast in my life before*, I thought, dully amazed that I was capable of such speed, catching the surreal sound of my feet thudding in a rhythm on the parquet flooring as the fear and the shame propelled me effortlessly forward down the long, empty corridor.

Maybe I can run for the school team, I told myself as I ran into the boys' toilets. *If I won medals, bet that would shut them all up!* I thought, locking myself in a cubicle and leaning, panting, against a graffiti-covered wall. *No more Cunt Fuck John then!*

The days of being called 'Blinker Boy', so shocking and wounding to me just months before, now felt like a lost time of innocence.

10

The Cupboard

Forget any learning, forget forging friendships. I realized very quickly that any chance of all that was out the window.

Within days of starting secondary school, I could tell that most of the teachers couldn't stand me. I was a pain in the arse to them, and my classmates started to think so too. Soon everyone – the whole school – knew who I was. I hated the attention, but it was impossible for me to avoid it. I provoked a reaction in people – pity, laughter, fury, violence – I could never just *be* with them.

School became a matter of survival for me. What could I do? I had no choice but to bear it. I became hyper-vigilant, not just at school but all day long, surveying every scenario for signs of danger, on the lookout to protect myself from harm.

My English teacher, Miss Jenkins, had a reputation for being the strictest teacher in school. I think she played on it, and – not that she ever smiled – I could tell that she enjoyed the power she had to intimidate.

I knew, minutes into my first lesson with her, that things between us were not going to progress well.

Small and tense-looking, everything about Miss Jenkins was neat: her brown bobbed hair, her navy suit and white pressed shirt; even the way she spoke was neat. She chose her words sparingly: said what she needed to say, then told us to get on with it. She was one of those very business-like teachers who were just there to get the job done as efficiently as possible, without any fuss . . . or enthusiasm or imagination, and definitely no joy.

No one liked Miss Jenkins, but they did what she said, because they were terrified of her. Her disciplinary skills were seen as exemplary by the school; new teachers were brought to sit in on her lessons, so they could see how it was done. Her classes were always deadly quiet: no mucking about, kids all working away, heads down.

Until she had me.

I was going to be a massive great big spanner in the works for her.

I was a reputation ruiner.

The fear and the dread that I felt about this keyed me up, and by the time I had my first lesson with her I was sweating from the outset.

Miss Jenkins was introducing the book we'd be studying, holding up a battered copy of something to the class. God knows what it was – I was too taken up with trying to contain the tics that were building up, hunched over, head down, grimacing with the effort of battling to keep them inside me. Nothing mattered to me more than this.

'*You*. Look at me when I'm talking to you.'

I can still remember Miss Jenkins's cold voice, the way she quietly strung out each word.

I looked up, just like she'd asked me to, but as soon as we locked eyes, a massive physical tic overtook me – as if all the tics that I'd been trying to hold back converged into one great spasm, like an electric shock – and sent me convulsing out of my chair.

'Stop this nonsense and sit back down.' She was almost whispering. When a teacher's confident enough to whisper, you know it's the right thing to be shit scared of them.

I sat back down. Then a tic sent me jumping back up again. Everyone gasped. I knew what they were thinking: *death wish*. I'd have been thinking that, too, if I'd been watching me.

She let silence hang in the air as I sat back down. 'I won't have anyone disrupting my class,' she said, fixing me with an unblinking stare. '*Do you hear me?*'

I did hear her, but hearing her didn't matter. Hearing her would only make things way worse.

Miss Jenkins was true to her word. She really wouldn't have anyone disrupt her lessons, and so she sorted it.

Next lesson, she told me to wait as I came through the door, then ushered me towards the book cupboard at the back of the class.

'Right, Mr Davidson, that's your cupboard now. In you go.'

I thought she was joking, but no – I could see a desk and a chair set up for me.

'You'll do your work in here from now on, OK?' she said. 'Until you learn to behave. Sit down and keep still. I'll be back to tell you what to do.' And she shut the door behind her.

A cramped, airless space with no daylight is not a place to sit when you're claustrophobic. I felt like I couldn't breathe, and I began to panic that I was going to pass out. I held on to the desk, taking long deep breaths, until Miss Jenkins opened the door again.

She was having me on, she was playing with me! I jumped up, ready to rejoin the class.

'Sit down!' she said. 'Listen! This is what the rest of the class are doing. I want you to write a poem in the style of Wordsworth.'

Who's Wordsworth? I had no idea.

'I'll be back at the end of the lesson,' she said, shutting the door.

Left alone again, with no one to judge me, I began to cry. Ever since I'd started at Gala Academy, I'd been trying so hard to keep my game face on, and it was exhausting. It was a relief not to care for a moment. Once I'd started, though, I just couldn't stop.

I didn't even attempt to write the poem.

Miss Jenkins gave me detention when she saw that I'd done nothing. I had to stay behind after school and write a hundred lines for her.

I must concentrate in class. I must concentrate in class. I must concentrate in class.

For every English lesson after that, the cupboard door was open for me.

I never did any work in that cupboard, so the detentions continued, and I had to write line after line after line.

I must sit still in class. I must listen in class . . . In the end, the lines were pretty much the only writing I did for Miss Jenkins, but still nothing changed.

If I was going to disobey her, she said, then I'd have to suffer the consequences.

She kept me there, doing nothing, learning nothing, every single lesson.

As the days passed, I became more and more withdrawn at home. 'What's the matter?' Mum said when I came back from school, my face all puffy and blotchy from crying.

'I'm just hot, that's all,' I said.

I couldn't tell her that a kid in the year above had hit me on the back of the head with a stone, and when I'd told him he was a fucking idiot, he'd gone and punched me in the face. There was no point; she was stressed out enough as it was.

Things with Dad and Mum weren't good. He'd even started eating his meals down the pub. His absence was never acknowledged, but Mum was all tense and rigid and snappy, and I could see she'd lost loads of weight.

Mealtimes had never been non-stop chat in our house, but they became weirdly quiet.

I took my family's silence as a communal seething anger, aimed at me. *This is all your fault*, they were saying. *He's not here because of you.*

Lately, a new tic had arrived, making mealtimes an upsetting time for all of us. I'd begun spitting out my food. This new silence made me anxious, and so I started up with it again, spitting out mouthful after mouthful. Everyone was pretty good at ducking, but one meal, William wasn't quick enough and I sprayed a mouthful of peas in his face. His yelling made me tic again – a jerk this time, making me swipe a fried egg off my plate.

'Enough!' Mum slammed her hands on the table. 'That's it, John. If you're going to behave like a dog, I'll treat you like a dog. Get down from the table, take your plate and eat on the floor with them,' she said, waving towards Bonny and Honey.

So I did. I put my plate next to Honey's bowl and sat down beside her.

When you're a kid, you normalize how things are in your family, don't you? Things are just the way they are, and that's that, so if I was upset by this, I don't remember it. It was my favourite meal, I do remember that – I always loved it when Mum gave us peas and chips with fried eggs – and I had to push the dogs off as I tried to get it down as fast as I could, to stop them from nicking the lot.

It was meant to be a punishment. Mum hoped it would bring me to my senses and make me eat properly again, which, of course, no surprises, it didn't. I actually preferred sitting there – the irony! I don't think she'd ever reckoned on that. But it was way more relaxing for me to sit on the floor, with my back to everyone and no one watching me, all tense and on edge as they waited for the next mouthful to shoot in their direction.

I shifted around a bit so I was facing the fireplace, and could direct my mouthfuls in there so Mum wouldn't need to fret about the state of her carpet.

Maybe I should be, but I can't even be angry with Mum.

I'd hear her going at Dad when he got back from the pub: *You've got to do something, David, you're not hard enough with him, you need to get that boy under control.*

There were no rules on how to parent in this situation. She was just doing her version of tough love, and I know it was a bit off the mark, but to be honest, that's what a lot of parents did back then.

11

Surviving It

Every day at school was an endurance test for me, but there were small things that kept me going. I even enjoyed some of the classes, anything that meant I wasn't required to sit still. It helped, too, that the teachers of those subjects were among the handful who were actually nice to me. Mr Moffat, my PE teacher, was one of them. I think he could tell I was trying, and he did everything he could to include me. If he saw me around school, he'd make a point of coming up to me.

'Are you OK, John? Is everything all right?'

'Aye, not too bad,' I'd say, even if things were anything but. It made such a difference to me, just knowing that someone was looking out for me and could tell I was struggling.

'Don't worry about those noises you're making,' he'd say in the lesson. 'It's not bothering me, or the rest of the class.'

I knew I was bothering the rest of the class, because kids at that age can't hide their disdain, but just knowing he was OK with it made me more relaxed when I did PE, and while nothing could stop me from ticcing, being less stressed meant the tics came a lot less often.

Mr Hill, who taught me DT, was another teacher who was unusually supportive of me. An older man, nearing retirement, he had a lovely, patient way about him, chatting away to me as we worked side by side. He was always checking in on me, too, never making a big deal of it, just casually enquiring after me once in a while.

'How are you feeling today, son?'

I'd be bent over, head down, concentrating on cutting the wood for my bird house, or pen holder, or whatever.

'Not too great today, sir,' I'd say. 'I've been struggling a bit lately.'

I found it much easier to be honest if I was doing something practical with my hands and not having to make eye contact.

'Aye, it must be hard for you, son, I can see that,' he'd say. 'Don't forget, now – what did I say? Measure twice and cut once. One more measure, go on, before you dive on in.'

'OK,' I'd say, 'I get you.'

'You just need to slow down. No rush, easy does it.'

Slow down. It really helped me to be taught how to do things in a more considered way. I'd always struggled with impulsivity, even before the Tourette's, but now it had become a real problem. I could see that when it came to being attacked in the playground or in the loos, or anywhere, my impulse to retaliate without hesitating only ever made things worse.

Over time I developed strategies to help me to cope. When the tics would get too much, I'd ask the teacher if I could leave the class to go to the toilet. Just getting away from the pressure of the classroom and walking helped me to calm down. Soon I'd find any excuse to leave. *I feel sick. Can I get a drink of water?* It was hard for the teachers to say no to things like that.

I was in the toilets one day, taking time out again, having a drink from the water fountain, when I felt a blinding blow to the back of my head. The force of it sent my face smashing into the metal bowl.

Standing up, I put my hand to my face to see blood streaming over my fingers. For a second all I could do was stand there numbly, staring at the blood, waiting for the pain to hit.

Titch Turnbull and Rob Hunter, two boys from the year below, were behind me, laughing their heads off, and they started shoving me, goading me for a reaction.

'Leave me the fuck alone!' The words came out slurry through my swollen lips. 'Look!' I said, swiping the back of my hand over my bloodied mouth. 'Look what you've done!'

They just carried on laughing. That enraged me. It was humiliating. They were younger than me. They were meant to fear me, or at the very least have some respect for me. This went so far against the natural order of things.

I lifted my hand and punched Titch square in the face.

He hit the deck, and Robert was gone before I'd even looked up.

'You did this to me.' My blood was spilling out on to Titch's shirt as he writhed on the floor. 'You deserved that, so make sure you fucking behave. Leave me alone in future, OK?'

His eyes had gone all massive and he couldn't speak. He just nodded as he scrambled to his feet and out the door.

I thought I'd put an end to being picked on. I really did. Nursing my sore knuckles, I was wobbly with the shock of it, but I didn't regret it. I was glad, relieved to have established myself as someone not to be messed with.

Then, later that day, I was hauled into the headmaster's office.

'What's this I hear?' The headmaster had this way of pulling back his head and looking down his nose at you, like he was really tall, even though he was about five foot eight, if that. 'I've been told you attacked Titch Turnbull and Robert Hunter for no reason.'

I explained as clearly as I could what had happened. I didn't even tic – the adrenaline kept me on track – and I honestly thought he'd believe me.

He dismissed me immediately. He'd be calling my parents, he said. I'd be staying behind for detention. *Let this be the last of this out-of-control behaviour from you, Mr Davidson, OK?*

Things became much worse in the playground for me after that. I think I was seen as even more of an easy target. The message had been given now that anyone could pick on me.

It was open season. Anyone could do what they wanted to me – hit me, spit on me, call me whatever – safe in the knowledge that if I dared to retaliate, it would only ever be me, not them, that got in trouble.

12

Darker Forces

The streets of Gala didn't feel like a safe place to be any more, either.

I'd had a run-in with a lass with a squint who drove the bakery van. She'd had a vendetta against me ever since I'd shouted out '*Cockeyed!*' at her. It hadn't landed well.

Every time she saw me now, she'd stop her van to holler 'I'm going to get you, you little bastard!' which only made me call her cockeyed again. True to her word, she did get me, too, running after me when she saw me cycling down Roxburgh Street one morning, pushing me off my bike and sending me flying in front of a bus. I just missed it by an inch.

She'd had it up to here with me, Mum said when I told her. She'd report it to the police, but from now on I had to stay away from trouble. I promised her I'd try. But what did that mean? Staying away from trouble just meant staying away from people, which isn't easy when you live in a town.

I worked out a back route to school, which took me out of town and away from the streets, through the fields. It added about half an hour to the journey, but it kept me away from anyone else.

Mum noticed the toll my new route was taking on my uniform, the rips in my trousers which I got from the hedges and scrambling over all the stiles, tutting as she got the needle out again. I needed to be more careful. She could only stretch to one set; I had to make it last, she said.

Every day, just the thought of walking through those gates got harder and harder. I'd be dragging my heels through the fields, trying to come up with some excuse to head home again. *Could I say I have a headache, one more time? Would she buy that?* I was wondering as I stood there in the last field before town, trying to work out how to get round a massive great sea of cowpats.

Oh my God, I thought, *Davidson, you're genius.*

'Thank you, if there is a God, thank you,' I said, down on my knees now, looking up at the sky. And then I lay down and I rolled in the cow shit.

I did it for as long as I could bear it, trying not to breathe through my nose as I coated my one and only blazer, and my one pair of trousers, making sure my shirt had some on it too, for good measure. *So sorry, I had an accident, Mum.* I practised what I'd say to her in my head. *I fell! I cannae go to school now like this, can I?*

And then I stood up and headed back home.

I was too much for Mum. I was wearing her out. (I was too much for both my parents, but Dad had voted with his feet, and we rarely saw him.) No one told me this directly – how much too much I was – but I'd got good at listening in from the top of the stairs, and I didn't need to earwig to see how much Mum was struggling.

My granny and grandad on Mum's side were coming round a lot more than they used to. Normally I would have welcomed this. All of us loved our granny and grandad – in a reverential, slightly-scared-of-them way. Now, though, their presence just served as an uncomfortable reminder to me that they were only here to help alleviate the stress of things – in other words, *the problem that was me*.

My grandparents were very proper, upstanding kind of people. I thought of them as posh; I think we probably all did. Always nicely turned out, in pressed, starched clothing, with never a hair out of place, everything about them was neat and clean, and they invested a lot of their time in keeping things that way. Grandad was forever washing his car, and not just washing, buffing up the paintwork till it shone. Fastidious – you know the kind of person I mean.

They had no time for hobbies, the two of them, because their house was their hobby. Weekends for them were a nonstop round of chores: window cleaning, dusting, hoovering, polishing, in their never-ending mission to keep mess and dirt at bay. They'd only take a break from this on a Sunday morning, when church became their priority. They were both active members, with Granny being especially involved. She was a church elder, in charge of flowers and stuff like that, which to me just added to her intimidating properness.

All church-going people were easily offended. Whether this was true or not didn't matter; I just had it in my head as a fact. Swear words were a no-go – that was definitely a given with my grandparents – and I knew this was true just from the way they'd gasp in horror if any of us kids said, 'Oh God,' because we must *never, NEVER, do you hear me*, they'd say, frowning, wagging a finger, *ever take the Lord's name in vain.*

They were kind people but their properness and my Tourette's made it harder and harder for me to be around them. So when my mum said I was going to stay with them, just me – *and isn't that a lovely, special treat, John? Aren't you lucky?* – there was no rush of excitement. All I could think was, *God – no, mustn't say 'God'. Fuck – no, do not on any account say that, either. Shit – no – how am I going to cope with this?*

Grandad knew that keeping me active and busy helped me to tic less, so I'd barely put my bag down before he had me up a ladder with newspaper and white vinegar, buffing up their front windows till they sparkled. At least when I was outside, Granny might be slightly less likely to hear me *fuck-fuckety-fucking*.

'Look, son.' Grandad was handing me up a bucket of soapy water, taking the dirty newspaper from me. 'I know you're having difficulty, you know, using these *bad words*.'

'Bad fucking words, cunt!' I ticced, making him wince like I'd squirted lemon in his eye.

'Exactly, yes,' he said. 'I just want to say that when Granny is around, the one word you do not ever use is . . .'

'Right,' I interrupted, thinking, *Oh no, I must not say the C-word, I must not, I must not. Don't tell me not to say it, please, don't tell me, whatever you do.*

Too late.

I felt that familiar tension, rising up from the pit of my stomach, when I saw Granny through the window, setting our cups of tea on a tray. The pressure mounted as I saw her coming out of the front door, all smiles.

'I've got you some tea, and some pink wafer biscuits,' she said, taking tentative mustn't-spill-one-drop steps towards us.

'Granny cunt!' I yelled out. 'Cunt granny!'

I remember how cold that sweat of shame felt on my forehead as I caught my grandad's sunken, disappointed face and watched him shaking his head in despair.

'John, we don't say that word.' Granny was trying to keep her voice even. 'It's a very bad word indeed,' she said, handing me my tea.

'I know, I'm sorry, CUNT!' I said. 'No! Sorry, so sorry, Granny' – shoving a pink wafer biscuit in my mouth to try to stop me from crying.

'I know it's not easy for you, but it's not nice to hear,' she said, 'and we don't do that here. We don't ever use bad words here, OK?'

I think she was genuinely hoping that my Tourette's could be location-specific, so it didn't need to happen at their house. *How could dirty language be possible in a place as clean as this?* I know how she felt; I often wondered that, too.

Grandad did his best to keep me working outside after that. Later that day he had me weeding the front flower beds, while he went to sort the brakes on his car.

I watched, fascinated, as he reversed out of the garage, then used a jack to lever the front of his car up, until there was enough room for him to lie underneath it.

Bored of weeding, I dropped the trowel and went to take a closer look. I crouched down next to the jack and touched it to try to make sense of how it operated. But I realized I needed to see it in action to fully understand, so I took the handle and started to turn it. Captivated by the feel of it, the pleasing effort of it, I didn't even notice the car lowering slowly, down and down.

It was the roar from under the car that made me stop, sending me falling back into the flower bed.

'What the fuck do you think you're doing?' my grandad yelled, his bright red face poking out from under the car.

'Sorry, Grandad, I'm so sorry, I didn't know, I didn't realize the handle did that!'

'Are you fucking joking, John?' I didn't like him yelling; he never yelled. 'What the fuck did you think it fucking did?'

Now there was a shriek from the open kitchen window.

'Language! Brendan, goodness me!' Granny was leaning so far out I thought she might tip right on to the grass. 'What on earth has possessed you?'

I remember just sitting there, in the damp soil of the flower bed, thinking, *I can't believe my grandad just swore*, having one of those moments you sometimes get as a kid, when you have to readjust your opinion of an adult and they suddenly seem just a bit less superior, and the order of how things are meant to be briefly goes all blurry and confusing before it shifts.

The next morning, my grandparents said it was time for them to drop me home again.

'But I thought I was meant to be staying for the week?' I said.

'No, no.' Granny had my bag packed and was putting it in the boot of the car. 'Just a day and a night – that's what we agreed. Come on now, John, hurry up. We can't leave until you put your seatbelt on.'

Back home again, I left them having a cup of tea with my mum in the kitchen and settled in on the top stair, with my head squeezed through a gap in the banister, so I could hear what they had to say about me.

'Heather, we can see what you mean.' My granny was talking. 'You're right: he can't help it,' she said.

'I'm so relieved you can see it,' Mum said. 'It helps me, you know, to know that you understand.'

'If you want my opinion,' Granny said, 'for what it's worth.'

'Go on, then,' Mum said.

'I wonder if it's because he's being possessed by darker forces.'

There was just this horrible echoey silence after Granny said that.

What did she mean? I heard the chink of a spoon in a mug, then an awkward cough from my grandad.

Do I have the devil in me? Is that what she's saying? I was staring at my hands, turning them over and over. *Wouldn't they be red, though, if that was the case?*

My mum has a massive set of lungs on her.

I bet the whole street heard exactly what she thought about that.

They probably gossiped for days about how Heather laid into her parents, screaming at them for talking a load of old nonsense. *About what, though?* They must have been dying to know – and concluding, I don't doubt, as we knew all too well already, that you never, ever, whatever you did, wanted to get on the wrong side of Heather.

13

822 727

The memory of what came next still feels like something out of a dream. Maybe because it began in the middle of the night, and I was bone tired – I remember that particular, heavy tiredness, which I felt all the time back then, which makes my memories blurred, like I'm looking back through a smeared, dirty window.

But it happened all the same.

I was twelve years old and didn't want to face it, but, bit by bit, my tics had been steadily increasing. The eye-twitches and jerks were still with me, and now there was barking to add to the roster, and grunting and the odd bit of yelping.

Oh yes, never a dull moment round ours.

I think my mum had started to worry that the neighbours would report her for mistreating her dog.

One night I barked, and the sound bounced off the walls and echoed round our tiny little downstairs bedroom.

Outside a dog barked back in reply, and a neighbour shouted to shut it up.

'John? Come on!' William moaned, his voice crackly with sleep. 'Will you give it a rest now?'

'I'm sorry, I'm sorry, Will.' I kept on apologizing, but it made no difference.

I barked again, even louder.

I don't recall the sound of the footsteps, or the door opening, but I remember my mum was suddenly there, in our bedroom, standing over me.

She looked like she was ten foot tall, and her face was all twisted and flushed with anger as she shouted at me.

'Mum, Mum, no!' I tried to wriggle from her grasp as she grabbed me by the hair and dragged me out of bed, but my scalp stung as she held on to me hard.

'I'm sorry!' I was yelling now. 'Just stop!'

But she couldn't, and she didn't.

Just like me, she couldn't stop.

I don't remember how we got to the sitting room, but the two of us must have stumbled in the dark up the stairs, clumsily joined together by her clenched fist and my hair.

I remember my eyes blinking in the brightness from the overhead light, and there we were: just me and my wild-eyed mum, looking at each other, like two boxers scoping each other out before a fight.

'John, I can't cope with this any more!' Mum was roaring.

'I'm so sorry.' I whispered it because it sounded so weak, and it was pointless – being sorry didn't make it stop.

'What is it?' she said, and for a second she didn't look mad with me, she just looked desperate and worn down. *What the hell is wrong with you?*

She seemed so scared in that moment, and noticing that fear in her eyes for the first time undid me, and I broke down.

She was my mum. She was meant to know the answers. *I* was allowed to be scared – I was just a kid, after all – but if she was, too, then it felt like game over to me.

'I dinnae know, Mum, I just can't explain it,' I said, my words gargled through my tears.

It was this, the not knowing, that made it so hard. The tics were bad enough, but the worst of it was that there was nothing definite, no plan of action.

'I want to die, Mum,' I said – *there you go, that was definite* – 'I wish I was dead.'

'Don't be stupid, John, what are you talking about?' she said, and now she was crying, too.

'I mean it,' I said. 'You'd be better off killing me.'

As an adult now, looking back, I hate that I said that to her. No parent should ever have to hear their child talk that way. But that's how desperate I was, and, given what followed next, you may actually think that I was right to be.

I couldn't tell what Mum was thinking now. Was she angry, or sad? Her face just looked blank, and her voice had gone flat like she was running out of battery.

'I want you to phone Dingleton Hospital,' she said, nodding to the landline on the wall.

I knew all too well what that meant.

Everyone knew about Dingleton Hospital. The name was bandied about in the schoolyard whenever anyone did anything stupid – which was all the time; we were twelve-year-old kids, after all, and hardwired for constant stupidity.

'Oi, you idiot, watch out – you'll end up being locked up in Dingleton!' was an all-too-familiar put-down.

It was the early eighties, and empathy for mental health conditions was thin on the ground – in the playground in

Galashiels, at least. Psychiatric hospitals were only ever known as 'nuthouses', and their patients were 'spazzes' and 'retards'.

That was me.

Mum's hand was shaking as she wrote down the number for me on a Post-it:

822 727.

Which, forty-odd years later, I still know off by heart.

'Dial it,' she said, patting her eyes with a tissue. 'Go on, you can speak to those doctors and tell them they're going to have to come and pick you up and get you sorted out.'

By now I was crying so hard I couldn't move, so she picked up the receiver and handed it to me, and dictated the number as I dialled it.

A woman answered the phone.

'Hello? Can someone come and get me?' I was hiccuping from all the crying. 'I need help, my mum says,' I said, swiping my nose.

'OK, can you tell me a little more?' She sounded kind and calm, like this was an everyday, normal kind of call for her, which I suppose, thinking about it now, it probably was.

'I don't know.' I looked up at the ceiling, staring at the white Anaglypta swirls, like icing on a cake, as I searched for the words.

'I think I've gone out of control,' I said.

14

Code Red

I didn't leave for the hospital that night.

'Go to bed now,' the woman on the other end of the phone had said, with her soft, soothing voice, like the bunny from the Cadbury's Caramel ads, 'and try to sleep. In the morning, go and see your doctor, and we can take it from there.'

Take it from there. The vagueness of that phrase. It could mean anything, couldn't it? From giving me a lobotomy – I wished I'd never watched *One Flew Over the Cuckoo's Nest* – to being wrapped up in a warm fluffy blanket in front of the telly.

I went with the warm-fluffy-blanket version that night, just so I could calm myself down.

I still wasn't OK, but not going straight to hospital made hope briefly rise inside me. *Maybe things are OK after all*, I told myself. *Me and Mum just got ourselves into a bit of a lather. It's late; things just got out of hand.*

'I'll be fine in the morning,' I whispered to myself as I got quietly, carefully, back into bed – mustn't wake William – 'everything's going to be fine by then.'

It felt like I'd dodged a bullet. I think I may even have slept a bit that night, but I dreamt of that bullet, travelling from the other side of the world, and in my dream I kept ducking and dodging, but it carried on in its trajectory – straight and clear and precise – as it moved in slow motion towards me.

The next morning, Mum and I took a taxi to the doctor's surgery. I remember the build-up on the journey, how serious it all suddenly felt. *We're in a taxi, and Mum's not speaking*, I told myself, my breath misting up a cloud on the window. *This is something big*, I thought, swiping line after line through the condensation, my finger squeaking along the glass.

My stomach swirled as we drove down the familiar streets of Gala. There was old Mrs Roberts crossing the road, with her wee sausage dog. My mouth was dry – I can recall that, and driving past Mr Hawkins waiting for the betting shop to open, fag in hand. When we arrived outside the surgery, I remember a dread overtaking me, draining me of all my strength, and feeling like my legs might just give way as I stepped out of the taxi.

There was something about going through that door that felt unbearable to me.

Mum had to push me through.

Tourette's is all about a lack of control – there's the irony – but still, I must have been clinging on to something, because as I walked into that surgery, I felt like I was losing the last bit of control that I had.

The waiting room was filled with elderly, proper-looking people, the kind that might easily take offence. I covered most of my face with my coat and put a hand over my mouth, pressing it down tight, but just a glimpse of a formally dressed woman reading *Good Housekeeping* was enough to make the words want to come.

'*BITCH!*' I muffled it in the lining of my parka and covered it with a follow-up pretend cough.

Mum didn't flinch. She sat there in silence, straight-backed and still, just staring at the clock on the opposite wall, without blinking.

We must have made for a weird-looking pair.

The sweat was dripping off me now – the coat over my face didn't help, but also from the sheer force of will and effort required for me to hold it together. It was sweat-making stuff.

The minutes ticked loudly by as we sat in that quiet room surrounded by strangers, with me writhing and sweating away in my seat as I tried all I could to keep a lid on it. The hand on the clock never seemed to move forward, I noticed, focusing on that now to keep me distracted. No matter how many times I checked, it looked like time had ground to a halt.

'John Davidson!' The doctor's voice made me jump in my chair, and I went red as I felt everyone's eyes on me.

'Come through, will you, please?' he said, beckoning from the doorway of his room, ushering us through.

Dr Robertson, as he introduced himself to us, was small and grey-haired, and carried himself with the confident air of someone who knew all the answers.

Mum sat down opposite him, but I remember just standing there. *I need to be standing for this*, I told myself. Sitting down felt like giving in.

'Sit down,' Dr Robertson said. So, of course, I did, in a heartbeat. He was a doctor. You did what a doctor said.

'How can I help?' he asked, in a manner that was both intimidating and reassuring at the same time.

We're in the hands of a professional. Oh God, I thought, and then, *thank God*.

And just like that, my mum started sobbing. *The shame of it.*

There she was, crying in front of Dr Robertson, in his room with all the big fancy books on the shelves, as he sat there behind his mahogany desk.

I don't know if it was the shock of it, or the shame of it, but now I was joining in, and we were both crying in front of him.

I wanted to apologize, but I'd been trying so hard to keep the words in as I waited that now nothing would come out when I wanted it to.

'It's OK,' he said, waving a box of tissues at us. 'Take your time.' He wasn't unkind, but he wasn't soft either. If it moved him to see two of his patients in such noisy, mucus-filled distress, then he definitely wasn't going to show it.

Mum had a go at explaining – as best she could through her raggedy crying – all the things that had been going on with me.

Dr Robertson listened, his face impassive but concentrating hard, holding a pen between his forefinger and thumb, poised as if ready to write.

'Well,' he said, when she was done. 'I think it's clear that we are at a crisis stage.'

Now Mum was crying even harder, and she was rocking with it, too. *Like a right loony*, I was thinking, wishing she'd get back to being Mum, the public Mum – *I mean, maybe it's her that needs to see a doctor.*

I just sat there, thinking about that, waiting for an emotion to come, but nothing arrived.

Crisis? What did that even mean for me? How was I meant to tell?

'I think the next step is admitting John to hospital,' Dr Robertson said, peering at us over the top of his glasses.

Mum nodded, looking down at the carpet, as she dabbed at her eyes.

'We just need to get to the bottom of what's going on,' he said.

I had an image of a deep-sea trawler when he said that, its net dredging up the murky seabed, and wondered, dully, what they might find at the bottom, wherever that was.

15

The Verdict

I didn't go back home from the doctor's. Can you believe it? I had no idea it could happen like that. I don't know what I'd been expecting: maybe a name for what was going on with me – that would have been good – and then, if I was lucky, some pills to make it go away.

Not hospital.

At some point I stopped listening to what the doctor was saying. I went into my head and concentrated my energy into trying to make the tics stay put inside me. Still, I could tell there was an urgency building in the room, just from the staccato way Dr Robertson was speaking, and how he kept chopping his hand on the desk to make a point.

My response was to squeeze my eyes tight shut, and to tic like crazy, because trying not to had made no difference. I was now yelping and twitching all over the place.

'This is obviously a serious situation,' I heard the doctor say, as I zoned out of my head and back in again. 'It's not tenable for you to live this way.'

'*Tenable!*' I ticced, repeating it again and again, because I didn't know what it meant, apart from not good, *definitely not good at all.*

Everything felt over my head.

I was drowning.

I thought of my last swimming test, the one when we'd all had to swim in our pyjamas, and the panic I'd felt as I was dragged down by the weight of them. *This is it*, I'd been thinking as I choked on the water, *I'm dead now*.

I'd wanted to be taken seriously for so long, but now it was finally happening, I didn't know what to make of it.

All those times Mum had been told she was a neurotic mother – *he'll grow out of it*, they said, *it's just a habit, nothing to worry about*. It should have felt like a victory now – or a massive relief, at least – but it didn't.

Careful what you wish for, I kept thinking.

It felt confusing, more than anything, to feel important, just not in a good way.

I'm an emergency.

'He's clearly had a full nervous breakdown,' Dr Robertson said, directing this at my mum. 'He needs to be admitted to the Peel General Hospital immediately. OK?' He gave another chop of his hand on the desk. 'OK, John?' he said to me, with a curt little nod.

It's not Dingleton, at least, thank God it's not Dingleton, I was thinking. 'Uh huh,' I said to the floor, because I wasn't brave enough to say, *No*. I wasn't confident enough to say, *Actually, I'm not sure what the hell you're on about. I've not had my lunch. Mum! You have to stop this, you have to say no! I'm meant to be watching the footy on the telly later – what if I'm not back for that?*

The term 'nervous breakdown' had always been a mystery to me, a catch-all phrase to cover all sorts, like when Janet Cole two streets down decided not to get out of bed – *nervous breakdown*, everyone whispered, knowingly – or when, out of the blue, Jason Heard started wandering round town without his kit on – *yep, a nervous breakdown for him, too.* He didn't look nervous to me; he looked quite pleased with himself, I thought. He didn't look like he'd broken down, either. The opposite, in fact; he was strutting down the high street, all full of himself, happy as Larry.

How did any of this relate to me? The words 'nervous' and 'breakdown' didn't add up to what I was feeling, but Dr Robertson had a great big massive desk, and all sorts of scary-looking medical instruments in glass cupboards behind him, and he sat up dead straight, like he knew he was the business, so I figured he must know his stuff. And anyway, what did I know? Lately, more and more, I'd been feeling like I didn't know anything. I didn't recognize who I was, let alone know myself.

And so nervous breakdown it was.

16

Taxi

Mum and I were standing waiting in reception for the taxi to take us to hospital. My hands were wet with sweat; they squeaked as I rubbed them together.

'How long do you think we'll be there, Mum?' I said as I gave them a good wipe-down on my trousers.

She didn't answer.

I had another go. 'An hour? Bit longer, maybe? The dogs will be wanting to be fed, that's all I'm thinking.'

It wasn't all I was thinking. I was thinking of injections and surgical gowns and a Victorian horror film I'd seen once where they'd performed an operation on someone without anaesthetic. *What will they be doing to me?*

'Don't worry about the dogs, John,' she said, all short and snappy-sounding. 'William's home – he'll sort them, won't he?'

I didn't think Mum looked herself. Her face had gone all blotchy, and she was blinking lots – big, flinching blinks – like the thoughts she was having were actually hurting the inside of her head.

'Come on,' she said as my shouts and twitches started up again. 'Let's wait out on the steps, shall we?'

The taxi, a blue Mondeo, was pulling up as we went

outside. I saw the leather jacket-clad elbow sticking out the window as it screeched to a halt in front of us, and when I heard Stray Cats playing at top volume, I knew straight away who it was.

'Keep your voice down when we get in, all right?' Mum hissed as Gerry, my dad's mate, greeted us with a double thumbs-up. 'You just know he'll be blethering about this to the whole of Gala, don't you?' she said from the side of her mouth.

'All right there?' Gerry said, with his wonky smile. 'How's it going?' His fag bobbed up and down as he spoke.

'We're very well, thank you,' Mum said as we got in the back. 'Everything's fine with us,' she added, waving away the fug of cigarette smoke and Old Spice with her hand.

Gerry had the biggest sideburns in Gala, and he wore his hair greased back and bouffed up with Brylcreem, like Elvis – well, a Gaelic version of Elvis, maybe. He was pale as milk and his hair was the brightest ginger.

'Is this an emergency?' he said. 'Do I need to be jumping the lights? You know me, eh, John?' He winked at me in the mirror. 'Any excuse.'

'No rush, thanks, Gerry. Just get us there safely, please,' Mum said, straightening her blouse, patting her hair down.

'What will they do with me in hospital?' I whispered to her, gripping on to the seat as Gerry took a corner way too fast.

'Oi, John! You fat bastard!' he yelled out to John Parsons, on the other side of the road. 'See you down the pub later, eh?'

'Language, Gerry, please!' Mum said. 'We're not fans of swearing in our house, thank you very much.'

'Sorry,' he said, grinning at her in the mirror. 'Forgot myself for a moment there.'

I rolled my window down so I could breathe a bit better through the smoke.

'Mum!' I tapped at her shoulder. 'I said, what will they do to me?'

She just shook her head and stared out the window, her cheeks all stripy from tears.

'I'm scared, Mum.'

'You'll be just fine,' she whispered. 'Don't worry now.' But she couldn't look me in the eye when she said it.

'What if it takes ages? I don't want you to leave me.'

'Shush now, don't say that, please.' And she repeated what Dr Robertson had said about getting to the bottom of it, and then she went dead quiet after that.

I hated it when Mum went dead quiet.

Gerry tried to crack jokes and chat to us to start with – he's one of those people who feel like they don't exist unless they're talking, I think – nice for a while and then exhausting. Anyway, he got the hint after a few of Mum's one-word answers, and entertained himself then by singing along to Showaddywaddy, loudly and off key, only stopping to shout out when he saw someone he knew.

'Mandy! New dress there? Looking good, looking mighty fi-ine!'

'Steve! You big' – pausing as he caught my mum's eye – 'mate, you owe me a fiver, don't forget now!'

It was a beautiful day. I remember squinting up at the clear blue sky and the sun shining bright, and thinking how wrong it looked, given my heart was racing so hard in my chest and feeling like it might burst right out of it. Storm clouds would be better, I thought, maybe with some thunder and lightning.

Fear was doing funny things to me. I was wearing my

favourite brown-and-cream patterned jumper and dark brown trousers, all 100 per cent nylon, so by rights I should have been boiling hot and sweating away like anything, but I was ice cold and shivering all over.

I'd never been to this hospital before, and I didn't know how to picture it. If there are gaps to be filled in, then my imagination goes into overdrive, and it's never something good that it fills them with. Now I was thinking of big white rooms, splattered with blood and littered with blunt-looking rusty implements. I groaned at the thought of it, and the groan morphed into a grunt and became a tic, and I grunted over and over, wishing that I'd never watched any of those Hammer horror films. *You'll regret it*, Mum had said when she'd caught me and my sister watching one, and she was right.

I wanted to open the back door of the cab. I could do a stunt roll out on to the road and then get up and run for my life. I could head to the river, or my granny's, or I could hide in the forest, up a tree. *No one would find me there.*

I had to force myself to think of Mum to make myself stop, and I pictured her slumped at the bottom of the stairs the previous night, head in her hands, crying and saying, 'I'm at the end of my tether.'

I'm doing this for you, Mum, I said to myself, taking my hands off the door handle, sitting tight. *They'll mend me, and then you can get back your tether.*

17

Apples and Bananas

When we arrived outside the hospital, I couldn't get out of the taxi. I just sat in the back, curled up tight so no one could move me. Mum tried to coax me out, calmly and quietly at first, keen, as always, to avoid a scene – *anything to avoid a scene*. I remember her whispering, pleading with me – *come on now, for goodness' sakes, John!* – as close to swearing as she'd ever get – *out you get!* – but I wouldn't. After a bit she got all high-pitched and upset, and she had to give in and call Gerry from the front to help her.

'OK, then, lad, out you get now.' He coughed, holding out a tobacco-stained hand, then yanking me out of the car. I was surprised by how strong he was for someone so skinny.

'Man up for your mum now, won't you?' he said, winding me with a too-strong slap on my back. 'They'll sort you out, and you'll be back home before you know it,' he added, 'right as rain.'

I closed my eyes as Mum grabbed me by the wrist and tugged me up the steps to the reception.

If I don't see anything, I kept thinking, *then it isn't happening.*

But inside, the smell made it all too real: l'eau d'hospital, that stomach-churning tang of methylated spirits and bleach, undercut with overcooked cabbage.

'Come on now, John, we're here now, pull yourself together,' Mum said.

I did my best, following her with my eyes only half shut now, as we made our way to the children's ward.

'I want to go home,' I whispered to myself as we passed porters pushing trolleys, and patients shuffling on their Zimmer frames. 'Soon I'll be home,' I said, passing visitors with bags of food and presents, bustling in and out, 'and it will all be over and done with.'

When I opened my eyes properly, we were standing in front of a tall woman with a paper nurse's hat perched on her short white hair.

'Hello there,' she said, with a quick, stretchy-mouthed smile. 'Please follow me.' And she was striding ahead of us already, down the long corridor, her rubber-soled shoes eerily silent on the shiny, polished floor.

'This is Dr Margerrison,' she said as she guided us into an office, where a young, fit-looking man was sitting, gesturing for us to join him.

I sat there, biting my lower lip tight, as he checked me over. I tried to keep myself calm to stop the tics from coming, as he listened to my chest and took my blood pressure, then shone a torch in my eyes.

What is he looking for? I pictured bright-green cartoon bacteria floating around in my eyes. *Catch them,* I thought, *just catch them and fix me, then hurry up and let me go.*

'Right,' he said, sitting back with a big, heavy breath. 'First and foremost . . .' *First and foremost?* I thought. *Who speaks like that? First and foremost, I want to get the hell out of here.*

'We are going to admit you to the hospital today, John.'

'Do you mean I'll be staying the night?' My voice came out squeaky high, like my sister's.

He nodded, and flashed a professional smile – *over and out* – to signal that was that.

'You'll be fine here.' Mum put her hand on my knee. 'You'll be safe. Come on, you're OK.'

I didn't like her talking that way to me, like she was expecting me to burst into tears. I wouldn't have that doctor thinking I was a pathetic cry-baby. *No way.*

'Yeah, I know I will,' I said, battling to keep down the horror inside me.

It wasn't just the fear of staying overnight, but even bigger: the fear of my fear being obvious, of showing myself up to the doctor.

'You know we can't go on like this,' Mum said.

'*Course.*' I gave a shrug. 'I know. I'm OK with it, aren't I?' I was too conscious of the doctor's quizzical gaze on me, like he was sizing me up, trying to decide if I was a wuss or not.

When had I last stayed the night away from my family? I cast my mind back and back and back, until I got to years ago, just that once, at Brendan Harris's house, when I was a wee little lad, when I was happy and easy-going, before any of this. *When I was nae bother to anyone.*

A nurse poked her head around the door.

'Would you like to come with me to look around the ward, John?'

Not really, no, I thought, but I nodded and smiled all the same, and followed her out, just to show the doctor I was fine. Still, I hated leaving Mum and him together, and fretted about them discussing me without me there.

Maybe the doctor knows what is wrong with me. I might have a rare, fatal disease that he doesn't think I'm ready to know about, and he's waiting for me to get out so he can tell Mum.

The nurse's name was Jane. She was lovely to me; I remember even relaxing a wee bit as she showed me round, introducing me to the children on the ward.

'This is David,' she said, gesturing to a small blond boy on a drip. 'He's been with us for a while now, haven't you, David?'

He smiled sleepily back at her.

I was scared by the sight of him. He looked so deathly white, and his face was huge, bloated from medication – steroids, as I later found out.

Poor lad, I was thinking. *Poor wee lad, what can be the matter with you?*

I wanted to say hi, I wished I could stay and chat to him, but Nurse Jane had moved on and I scuttled after her gratefully, eager to put some distance between me and the boy as fast as I could, because I could feel the word coming, climbing up my throat.

'Fatty!' I coughed into my hand. 'Fatty!' I coughed again, my cheeks prickling with the shame of it. *Sorry, so sorry, mate,* I thought as I looked back at him, far enough away now not to have heard me, but a relief, all the same, to see his eyes closed.

'Come and meet the wee bairns, John,' Jane said at the line of cots along the end of the room. 'You can help me out with feeding them one day, if you like. I can show you how to give them a bottle,' she said, bending down to pick up a cute, curly-haired girl, stretching out her arms towards her.

One day? How long does she think I'm staying for?

'Sorry, Jane, but I think I'm only here for tonight.'

'Oh, John, you'll be with us a wee bit longer than that,' she said, gently, as she jiggled the little girl.

I think my face must have shown what I was thinking, because she put the baby down and gave my shoulders a squeeze. 'It's OK, don't panic. It's a lovely ward, don't you worry.'

'Would it help to sit down?' she asked as my tics started up in a new and novel way. Now I was banging the end of the cot, whacking it, hating myself for doing it but not being able to stop. 'Why don't you have a rest?' Jane said, leading me back across the ward, as I kept on banging anything I walked past – a chair, a bed, a trolley – until she sat me on a tiny wee chair, outside the office where Mum was with the doctor.

'I can't cope any more, even on my medication,' I heard Mum say.

The doctor's voice was low, and he mumbled something in reply, but Mum's voice was high and shrill, and way easier to hear than his. 'His tics are getting so much worse . . . his behaviour is changing . . . he's not sleeping . . . he's refusing to go to school . . . he keeps complaining of pain, in his arms and legs . . .'

It was all true, what she was saying, but I hated hearing her talking about me, summing me up like that, making me sound like a nightmare.

'I wish I could assure you, Mrs Davidson, but, as I've said, I've not come across anything like it before. None of us have.' The doctor must have been standing up now, next to the door. 'We'll try him on some different medications, keep testing him, see if we can find some answers – OK, then?'

That was her cue to get going, but my mum just wailed.

Like an animal. Like my dog sounded once when it got caught in a rabbit trap in the woods.

I pictured the doctor, with lots to be getting on with, checking his watch, not knowing what to do with this woman sitting there in front of him all blotchy-faced and red-nosed and out-of-control hysterical. *She shouldn't be behaving like this, showing me up like nobody's business.*

My tics went into overdrive, and I started jerking and barking louder and louder.

The kids that had been sleeping were all awake now, looking at me wide-eyed from their beds, in the way that kids do when they're wee and don't yet know not to stare.

'*Stupid bitch!*' I shouted, then clamped my hand over my mouth.

'Sorry,' I said. 'Oh no, I'm so sorry about that.'

Everything had gone quiet. My mum in the office. The doctor. All the kids. There was just the *beep, beep, beep* of a machine.

Nurse Jane wasn't looking so smiley now as she hurriedly walked towards me. 'OK, John, that's not a nice word, now, is it? That's not OK.'

'Sorry,' I said. 'It just came out. I didn't mean it.'

'Well, can you try not to?' she said. 'There are wee bairns here and that's not good for them to hear now, is it?'

I shook my head, too worn down to even try to explain.

I'd expected it to be different in the hospital. I'd thought medics might be more understanding. But the nurse didn't get it, which made me worry now that maybe none of them would: the fact that I just couldn't control it.

'Why don't I take you to where you're going to be staying

tonight?' she said. 'How about that?' Her voice was sunshiney bright now, like a children's TV presenter.

I followed her, head down and silent, to a small glass cubicle at the end of the ward.

'This is where you'll be for tonight,' she said, patting the bed. 'Lucky you – you get your own special place!'

I wasn't stupid. I knew it was just to keep me from disturbing everyone.

I looked out into the ward and every child was still staring at me, and it felt even worse to be in the cubicle – more exposing, like I'd been put in a goldfish bowl.

'Right, I'll leave you to it,' the nurse said. 'I expect your mum will be in in a moment to say goodbye.'

I nodded at her, and smiled, trying to fool her because I was all set to go. Mum would listen to me; she'd get it, that there was no way I'd be staying.

I caught sight of the curtains as she left, and then yanked them shut, all the way around, so now nobody could see me.

Mum came in to say goodbye with the doctor. She gave me a hug, and she was trying to be all positive now in a formal kind of way, because of the doctor, who was hovering, looking like he needed to get going.

'I'll be here with Dad later,' she said, patting my hand. 'As soon as he's back from work with the car.'

I'll be getting straight in that car when you leave, I was thinking. *There's no way you're keeping me here.*

'We'll come with your pyjamas, and your washbag,' she said, 'and we'll bring you some fruit, you know: apples, oranges, grapes and bananas' – listing them all off, like I was a wee kid and didn't know what fruit was.

I don't need to cry, I thought as I watched her leaving. *She'll be back soon with Dad and the fruit, then I can go.*

I got straight into the bed when she was gone, and pulled the covers over my head, which had started hurting from the pressure of it all.

I can let a few tears out, I told myself, *now that there's no one here to see me.* And I started sobbing and couldn't stop.

I kept thinking of all those apples and bananas she'd be bringing me – I was mad about fruit back then – but even that didn't make me calm down.

It was the not knowing. I was just so tired of not knowing what comes next.

18

Diagnosis

No one knew what was wrong with me. That was the hardest thing for me to deal with – harder than being stuck in the hospital, away from my family, harder than being woken up and prodded and injected and experimented on all the time. I just wanted some proof – anything – to put an end to this. *Make it stop.*

It was frightening to be so alone with it. This thing, whatever it was, had taken me hostage – *couldn't anyone see that?* – and it felt like no one was coming in to rescue me.

Every single test they did came back negative. I kept waiting for the next result, ever hopeful at first, but gradually less and less so.

Nothing came up on the X-rays. The chromosome tests were all good. No, I hadn't got epilepsy. No, there were no abnormalities on my brain. No, no, no. *Maybe this will be the one*, I'd think, wincing as the needle went in for another blood test. *This could be it*, I'd tell myself, to keep myself strong, to stop myself feeling queasy – I'm squeamish like that – keeping my eyes tight shut so I didn't have to – *please God, no* – see my blood.

'Calm down!' I never got used to being told this by the doctors and nurses. It stung like a slap, every time. What they meant was 'control yourself', which just showed that none of them believed me, even though I told them again and again: *I can't help it.*

'Calm down,' they kept saying, not noticing that it made no difference, that it was worse than pointless, in fact. In the end, 'calm down' became a trigger for me to tic. *They're cross with me; I mustn't make them angry*, I'd think, and the stress of trying not to cause offence would set off a reaction inside me, making offence the inevitable thing.

You know that scenario you can find yourself in where there's a certain something you just mustn't say? *Don't mention the war* – that kind of thing – and your mind just keeps reminding you of it, the thing that you mustn't, at all costs, mention? And all that does is make you want to say it? And usually, thankfully, you don't, and you can breathe out again, relieved that all your internal panic was for nothing.

My panic was never for nothing, and it was pretty much constant now, because lately, since being in hospital, my tics had progressed again and developed a new subset to challenge me: *whatever the worst thing that must not be said is, I must say it.* I didn't think anything could be worse than swearing, but this top-trumped swearing every time.

'Fatty!'

She was a lovely nurse, one of my favourites, and maybe a little bit overweight.

I made her cry. I wanted to die when I saw her scurrying off across the ward, head down, trying to hide her tears. Then I pulled the covers up and had a cry, too.

I'm so sorry. I can't help it. I can't fucking help it. As time went on, I stopped saying it, and just kept these thoughts in my head. What was the point in telling anyone, explaining again and again, when it made no difference at all?

Calm down, calm down, calm down.

There was something about not being believed that made me feel a very particular, angry kind of loneliness. My rage and frustration mounted as the days passed and still nothing changed. I began to feel increasingly isolated from everyone, going inside myself more and more, and talking a lot less. I found it hard enough as it was to express my feelings, and I'd keep all those thoughts to myself, trying to bury them deep down inside me.

'Cunts, the lot of you!'

I did say I tried.

At a loss, the doctors kept trying me on all kinds of different medications, in the hope that something, one day – you never know – might do the trick. I didn't have epilepsy, but they tried me on epilepsy drugs. Nothing made me stop ticcing, but they all made me sleepy, which after a while I didn't mind. At least I didn't tic much when I was sleeping, and it was better, in a way, to sleep through things. *Wake me up when it's all over*, I kept thinking.

Eventually they settled on the drug haloperidol, a powerful antipsychotic. It knocked me out and I slept most of the day, staying in my corner cubicle with the curtains closed. I didn't want anyone to see me.

The doctors were saying I needed to see a psychiatrist, and that terrified me. It made me think of Dingleton Hospital again. *Perhaps I'm fucking mad*, I kept thinking. *Maybe they're going to lock me up in there for the rest of my life.* I was a twelve-year-old boy, though; I couldn't express this to anyone. The fear of it felt too big to let out. *If I say it, it might make it true,* I kept thinking. I'd just wear myself out with crying until I fell asleep.

What will become of me? That thought plagued me as I fell asleep, whirling around in my head without any answer to stop it.

It happened gradually, so slowly that I didn't even notice, but after a few weeks I became institutionalized. I hated being in hospital, but it became the only place in my whole world where I felt comfortable and safe. My cubicle became my little bubble. Now whenever someone approached to speak to me, I'd be overwhelmed by anxiety. *I don't like this, I don't like this,* I'd tell myself over and over, and I'd hide under the covers, hoping they'd go away and leave me be.

Mum came to see me in hospital every day or two. She looked so worn out and sad.

'Come on, son,' she'd say. 'You need to get up and move about. Let's get you something to eat at the cafeteria.'

At first I'd say no when she suggested this – I always wanted to avoid being in a public place if I could help it – but soon I was so drugged up it didn't really bother me. Nothing bothered me much any more.

The hospital cafeteria was huge and noisy, and the smell of overcooked mush permeated everything. About three months after I'd become a patient, I remember heading to the cafeteria with her. There was only one sticky table free in the corner, and Mum led me towards it, like I was a toddler who might get lost. The drugs made it hard for me to think straight. They made it hard for me to think pretty much anything.

I remember us sitting there, and Mum looking awkward, which she often did because it was so hard to have a conversation with me. My mind felt like sludge and I had to dredge up words, try to scrabble around in my head to pull out a sentence. Sometimes it was just too hard, and I'd give up and say nothing. Mum stopped trying too, after a while, and we sat there in silence as I attempted to force down a limp cheese-and-tomato sandwich.

'Shite food!' I yelled, spitting out a mouthful.

Mum wiped off the spray of breadcrumbs from her top.

'Wankers! You're all wankers!' I shouted.

I was used to the shocked faces and the stunned silence, but Mum never was.

'Come on, son.' She was standing up now, brushing the last of the breadcrumbs off her skirt. 'Let's get you back to the ward.'

'Excuse me.' It was the man on the next table. 'I couldn't help noticing . . .'

'Yes, sorry about my son,' my mum said – she was always quick to apologize for me. 'He's not well; that's why he's here.' She was in a hurry to leave now, grabbing her handbag, giving the mess I'd made on the table a cursory swipe with a paper napkin.

'No, no need to apologize, please.' The man was standing up now. He was in his thirties and smartly dressed, with that confident, assured air I'd come to associate with doctors.

'I'm just interested in what's going on with you.' He was looking at me.

'We don't know.' Mum was itching to get away from him. 'The doctors are looking into it,' she said, trying to lead me by my hand to the lifts.

'I'm a doctor,' he said, 'from Manchester.' Suddenly he was ahead of us. 'What floor are you on?'

Mum muttered a reply and looked around, eyes darting, all antsy and agitated.

'Great,' he said, pressing the button. 'I'm going to come with you – do you mind?' And he was in the lift before she could answer, beckoning for us to come in. 'I'd like to chat to your consultant, if that's OK?'

'I don't think that's necessary, but thank you.' Mum had her pinched look about her. 'He's already got the doctors helping him.'

'I'm a neurologist,' he said.

That did it – now he had Mum's full attention.

'OK?' she said. Anyone with an '-ist' after their name impressed her.

'I think – in fact, I'm certain – I know what this is,' he said as the lift doors opened on our floor.

He didn't get out immediately, but held the door to stop it from shutting. 'It's a condition called Tourette's syndrome,' he said.

I remember repeating those words in my head, over and over, as we followed him through the ward, and thinking how weird my face felt, and realizing it was because I was smiling, for the first time since God knew when – such a crazy long time – for the first time ever, it felt like.

19

The River

That first year after diagnosis, when I turned from twelve to thirteen, feels more like it lasted ten years in my memory. It's all hazy and blurred and chopped up, just a mash-up of stays in hospital – weeks on end at a time – and then weeks back at home, with a wee stint at school, and then back to hospital I'd go again. I can't remember which part came when, because time kind of lost its linear quality, thanks to the cocktail of medications they kept prescribing for me, chopping and changing after the latest combination had seemed to do nothing, or made things worse, or sedated me too heavily to function.

I was put on anticonvulsants and antipsychotics and antidepressants when I first came out of hospital. They just chucked all the antis at me, tweaking them when I'd go back for another stay – *let's try this one instead, we'll up the dose on that, maybe this combination will be more effective* . . .

There was so much that the doctors didn't know, and what strikes me now is their lack of curiosity. Only later, when I joined the Tourette's Support Group,* did I find out about the specifics of my condition – that there are different

* This became Tourette Scotland in 1994.

categories of Tourette's, and the particular kind that I have, with its coprolalia (swearing), echolalia (repeating words), OCD and ADHD, is known as Full-blown Tourette's Plus, which is basically as severe as it gets. But for now, it felt like I was just seen as this kid with this mysterious syndrome who upset everyone, and they just needed to find a way to shut me up.

Mum must have felt so alone with it all, when I think back to it now. She and Dad were barely speaking by then, and getting me to the appointments and making all the decisions, agreeing to this drug and *OK then, not that one* – that was all down to her. There was so much for her to manage. I think I was too drugged up to notice or even appreciate just how much she did for me at that time.

In the end, I just stayed on the antipsychotic haloperidol, but even on that I was bone tired and aching all over, and all I wanted to do was sleep. My speech was slurred, my mouth was dry, and the weight kept piling on.

Who knows? Maybe I could have taken all that if it had meant my symptoms disappeared, but it felt like I was ticcing as much as ever.

Was this it? Was this how life was going to be from now on?

The doctors couldn't give us any assurances either way.

I tried my best to stay positive. I really did. I remember dragging my sluggish limbs back to school, literally trying to put one foot in front of the other.

Stand up tall! Hold your head up! I told myself, thinking, *this is the very last thing I feel like doing right now*, but scraping that barrel all the same. *At least, finally, things will be better*, I thought, *now there's a name for it*, convinced that everyone would definitely be more accommodating and understanding when they knew I had a condition.

Ah, you've got Tourette's, have you? So sorry, mate, I had no idea. I shouldn't have been such a prick towards you. That kind of thing.

I wasn't prepared for the reality. In films and books, there's usually that point in the story, isn't there? When the people who do wrong, the 'baddies', either get their comeuppance or realize the error of their ways, then feel so bad, so eaten up by their behaviour, that they transform into better people. I thought that would happen – naive and hopeful as I was, I think I fully expected it – but this was one of those moments when the harshness of real life hit me full in the face. Of course it didn't go like that.

No one had heard of Tourette's. The name meant nothing, so for some pupils, now that I had *something*, all it did was give them another excuse to call me a weirdo, a freak, or a perv – it was official now! *Game on!*

After that, I was treated worse than ever.

I'd been back at school a few days, after my first stay in hospital, when my biology teacher, Mr Wainwright, lost his patience with me.

'Mr Davidson,' he said, banging his hand down hard on the desk, 'up the front you come.'

I forced myself out of my chair, clasping my hands tight together to hold back the twitching as I made my way up to the front.

'Right!' he said, with this strange, unamused smile he wore when he was taking pleasure in something that wasn't remotely funny.

'I want you to explain to the rest of the class why you're making these strange animal noises.' He'd pulled out a stool and was beckoning to me to stand on it.

Here it was: the opportunity for me to explain myself, unintentionally being handed to me on a plate.

'I have this condition, sir,' I said, clambering up, then forcing myself to look up from the floor, standing with my back ramrod straight. I wanted to look proud, show them finally I had nothing to hide.

I told them about the Tourette's, what it was, how it meant – as I'd been saying all along – that I couldn't help it, but my words were increasingly drowned out, at first by a few giggles, which soon morphed into full-blown laughter.

'Mong!' someone shouted out, mortifying me into silence mid-sentence.

'Well, if you can't explain it properly, Mr Davidson' – Mr Wainwright's smile was wider than ever – 'then it looks like I'll have to do it for you. It seems that Mr Davidson is a bit of a mad-head,' he said, playing to the laughter now, holding out his hands to welcome it. 'I think we've got a bit of a lunatic on our hands, don't you?'

That's the first time I remember experiencing blind anger. I felt no fear, no humiliation, no uncertainty, just a pure white rage, eclipsing everything, as I jumped down from the stool and pushed Mr Wainwright out of my way.

Running out of the classroom, all my heaviness and lack of coordination was obliterated, and I was nimble and light and fast, and briefly I felt invincible.

Anger can be really handy like that.

*

No one was in when I got back. All I wanted to do was curl up in bed, but I knew Mum would be back from work any minute now, and she'd hate it – she'd go nuts to see me here, back home in school time, yet again.

What did I say, John? What do I keep telling you? You have to stand up to them! Grow a thick skin!

She always said the same thing, and I'd always think the same thing:

You have no idea. This is too much for anyone. You couldn't deal with it, believe me, no one could.

I grabbed my fishing rod and headed to the river, to a spot where I knew no one would be.

The spot I went to was always dead quiet. I don't think anyone but me could ever be bothered with the assault course you had to endure before you got there: the tangle of brambles you had to push your way through, then the wet, slippery, rocky bit you had to scramble over next to get down to the water.

I was still in my school uniform – there was no way I could have changed out of it and left it for Mum to see I was skipping school again. I didn't care that I was trashing it. No matter that I'd just ripped a trouser leg on a thorn; fine by me that my school shoes were now caked all over in mud. I hated my uniform. I wanted it ruined. I couldn't stand any reminder of school.

The sky was grey and flat with a thin wash of cloud. At the edge of the bank, I put my rod down, and stood looking into the depths of the river. The water was clear and brown, like a weak tea before you put the milk in. It didn't glitter like it did on the sunny days, but it was clearer than ever, and I could see everything: the neon-green algae swaying in the current, minnows and bullheads darting in and out of the rocks.

Usually, I'd get that buzz and be all jittery and excited, scoping out the best bit to cast my rod, wondering where those big fish were hiding from me.

I sat down on a damp rock and waited for the buzz to happen, but it didn't come. Instead, a terrible heaviness overtook me.

I'm so tired of this, I told myself, pressing my fingers to my temples, *I'm just so fucking sick and tired of it all*, as I was bombarded with worries, all jostling for my attention.

Mum and Dad will be splitting up because of me, I told myself, *my family are all miserable because of me* – picking up a stone, rolling it around in the palm of my hand – *no one can concentrate in class, and that's my fault*, I thought, *I'm ruining everything* – chucking the stone in the water, watching the rings of concentric circles widening out around it.

I'm that stone, I thought, *affecting everyone and everything around me*. I stared at the ripples, expanding and flattening, till they were gone.

I don't even remember getting up. I don't remember the shock of the cold as I stepped into the water, or how the rocks felt under my feet, or how I got myself waist-deep. I just remember thinking, *It would be easiest to end it here, where it's quiet. All I want is some quiet.*

It *was* quiet, I remember that; even the water flowed silently around me as it kept pulling me and pulling me along with it.

Just do it, I told myself, *jump forward, put your face in*. And so I did.

The current is always strong along that stretch of the river. I floated face-down, dimly aware of how fast I was moving, as I waited for the sinking to start.

Sink, come on, sink! I kept saying in my head, as I was swept along on the surface.

I wasn't sinking, though.

The water was shallower now, and my stomach and knees were scraping along the riverbed. *This isn't working too well*, I thought as the current bundled me up in the shallows and the force of the water ejected me, spluttering and coughing, on to a shingle-covered stretch of riverbank.

I sat there for half an hour or so, in a hunched-over heap, with tears trailing hot paths down my frozen cheeks, only staggering to my feet when the shivering got too much, when it felt like my whole body was being powered by a vibrating motor.

I'm an idiot, I berated myself as I squelched my way back home. *I can't even kill myself*, I thought, stopping to take one shoe off, and then the other, tipping out all the water. *What kind of idiot fucks that up?*

I'd been poaching salmon and fallen in, I told my horrified mother as I stood in the doorway, dripping wet and shivering still, coated all over in weed.

She took me straight to the doctor's – in case I had a chill, she said – but then said she wanted to talk to him in private. She knew. And she knew that I knew she knew, too.

It was always unspoken between us, the thing that I tried and failed to do that day. Maybe it was just too sad and big to bring out into the open, without anything to hand to offer any solace, with nothing to be done, nothing to be said that could make things any better for me.

I had a chaperone at school after that, a teaching assistant, who would follow me around and check up on me in the playground, to see if I was OK.

I'd always try to find ways to stretch out our conversations, asking her anything about her life – her pets, her kids, what was she going to cook for tea tonight? – desperate to keep her talking. For as long as she was with me, I could stop looking over my shoulder and stand anywhere I wanted, instead of hovering next to the door, primed and ready to run.

20

Mint Choc Chip and a Packet of Bensons

So, now what? Mum was desperate to find us some help after I got diagnosed. I remember her being a bit frantic, phoning the doctors all the time, trying to get her hands on any kind of advice or information. *Are there any organizations? Numbers to call? Anyone who could help us at all?* She's always been like that – with this dogged determination – and it paid off when she discovered the Tourette's Support Group.

That first meeting we went to in Dundee was nerve-racking. I had no idea what to expect as we sat down in a group of about twenty folk with Tourette's, some of them kids, some adults, all of them ticcing away.

Bit by bit I started to let my guard down, taking it all in, and I could see Mum starting to ease up, too, her hands loosening in her lap. And I remember feeling a kind of stillness – which was weird, I guess, given all the noise – and thinking, *Thank you, thank God*. I was surrounded by people like me, and for once I didn't feel on my own.

There was something else I noticed, too – something I hadn't expected. Looking around at everyone's tics, the way they moved and shouted and blinked, no two tics were the same. Everyone's Tourette's was different. Mine included. I wasn't just different – *I was unique*. I think that felt better to me somehow, easier to live with.

The group became a regular thing for me and Mum. We'd go to the monthly meetings, no matter where they were in Scotland. In those early days after the diagnosis, I think the group meant more to her than me. She seemed more sure of herself, more confident in how to deal with me. She picked up some coping strategies there – stuff to try when I didn't want to go to school, after another spell in hospital. *I'm too knackered today, Mum; I've got a sore tummy; so sorry, I fell in cow muck again.*

The more she learnt, the more patient she became. And on the hard days – the ones when I just wanted to shut everything out – she was less likely to lose it with me.

'What else are you going to do with your time, John?' she would say, holding out a shopping bag for me. 'Rot in your bedroom all day long? Come on, remember what they said in the support group? You need to face things, not hide away. It's good for you to get out; you'll feel better once you've done it.'

I didn't agree. Every trip into town was an exhausting ordeal for me. It must have been for Mum, too, so hats off to her, because she kept on forcing me out with her even so. Every time there'd be some kind of drama – most often in the supermarket, which was only ever guaranteed to set me right on edge. I hated its harsh overhead strip lights, buzzing ominously away above me. I was in the spotlight, that's what it felt like, which made me more self-conscious than ever.

I couldn't stand the stark layout of the place, either; those long, shiny-floored aisles really intimidated me. I didn't like having to walk down them – on and on and on, it felt like – towards the other people, all watching me, or that's how it seemed to me. I felt too much on show; there was nowhere to hide.

The neatness and order of everything made me tense, the way all those packets of Frosties were stacked in a row, lined up and waiting, challenging me to knock them all off the shelf. I had to grab my wrist, to try to stop myself from giving them a good bashing. It didn't always work – sometimes my hand would fly out and I'd whack them, so they scattered and slid all over the floor. There'd be a right old fuss then. An outraged shopper would have a go, ask me what I was playing at, and I'd be down on my hands and knees saying, 'Sorry, sorry, I didn't mean to,' trying, all sweaty and red-faced, to gather them up as fast as I could, so I could shove them back – never as neat as they once were – on the shelf again.

If I wasn't knocking things off shelves, I'd be shoving old ladies from behind with my shopping trolley, or whacking Mum in the face.

'Shame on you! Don't you do that to your mother!'

Strangers would butt in to lay into me. Sometimes they'd lay into Mum, too:

'What kind of mother lets her son do that to her? Don't you discipline him?'

Mum found it easier to respond to them now that I had a diagnosis, at least.

'He can't help it,' she'd say. 'He has a condition called Tourette's syndrome.'

I don't think most people had even heard of it, let alone knew what that meant back then. Maybe the fancy French name and the word 'condition' was enough to stop them in their tracks. Perhaps it was Mum's icy, 'don't mess with me' stare. But for whatever reason, they'd usually back off.

I was fourteen now, and I remember a Friday afternoon, nearly the weekend, when I'd somehow talked Mum into letting me have the day off school.

'Just this once,' she'd said, 'since you've been good lately, going into school without any carry-on.'

She still didn't know that most days, after I went in, I'd sneak off at first break and spend the rest of the day in the woods near by, sleeping till it was time to head home. School must have known, but no one ever said anything to her. To be honest, I think I did them a favour – no more hassle, no more disruption in class. It was just easier for everyone that way.

So there I was, in the supermarket, helping Mum with the weekly shop.

She'd just sent me off to find a pack of Findus Crispy Pancakes, and I was in 'head down, no eye contact' mode, which seemed to be the best way to keep me out of trouble, even if it did make it tricky to work out which aisle I was in.

'Hey, John?'

My stomach did a flip when anyone said my name in public these days, and I gave a tentative sideways glance behind me, wary that a punch might just be coming my way.

It was Kevin – *thank God* – the dad of a lovely wee lad, Peter, whom I'd got to know in hospital.

'Hey there, Kevin, *you bald twat!*' I ticced.

'Good to see you, too,' he said, smiling. 'Not at school, then?'

'Aye.' I nodded.

'Not well?'

'Something like that, aye. How's Peter doing?' I said, changing the subject.

'Aye, you know how it is,' he said. 'He's never too good, but not too bad either, as it goes.'

'He's a good wee lad,' I said. 'Will you tell him from me I said hi?'

'Aye,' he said. 'He'll be made up when I tell him I saw you.'

Peter was a severely disabled boy I'd got to know in hospital. He'd come in for a few days at a time, so his parents could have some respite. I used to look forward to his stays – he was such a cheery wee trooper, and we formed quite a bond over the months. I knew how to make him laugh; he liked me singing to him and joshing about.

'Now, I'm just having a think to myself here,' Kevin said, 'and I'm wondering, might you be wanting some work, John?'

I couldn't believe that he'd asked me. I think I just looked at him with my mouth open.

'I could do with some help in the ice-cream van,' he said. 'Only if you're interested, like,' he added, to fill the awkward silence as I scrabbled around in my head, trying to work out what the right answer was.

Will I fuck it up? Will it make my tics worse?

'Yes!' I said. *Was that a tic?* I wasn't sure. 'Cheers, Kevin, I'd love to.'

That's it. I've done it now.

'Grand,' he said. 'Can you start tomorrow evening? I'm doing the rounds in the van. I could pick you up at six and I can teach you on the job as we go.'

I couldn't sleep all that night for fretting. My mind was whirring with terror and excitement, with the terror mainly winning out. I couldn't believe that Kevin – *Kevin!* – had asked me to work for him. *What was he thinking? Why did he think I could do it?*

This was a really, really big deal, and I didn't know whether that was a good thing – the bigness of the deal – or a bad thing, or rather, a *bad for me* thing.

Kevin and his special, home-made ice creams were properly famous round Gala, which may as well have been the universe to me then. He was like a celebrity, thanks to his ice creams, which were the best for miles and miles – and I'm talking absolute top-of-the-range quality, high end, here. What made them extra special was the fact that they were made to a top-secret recipe, which just added an extra layer of mystery and intrigue and made everyone chatter and marvel about them.

Kevin didn't just have a van; he had an ice-cream shop, too, otherwise known as a parlour, and just the word 'parlour' made it seem so super-fancy and exotic. I was in awe of his success and his reputation. Everyone in Gala knew who he was, *but in a good way*. Not like me.

It turned out all my fretting was for nothing, because I took to working in that van with such ease, and with a confidence that I hadn't realized I still had in me. There was something about being high up, and set above people, that made me feel safe, I think, and I could relax a bit when I realized people were less likely to see and hear my tics. I'd be still ticcing away – *fuck this, fuck that* – and my motor tics were going off, too, all the jerking and stuff, but nothing so severe that it would get in the way of what I was doing. People didn't seem to see them as much, and the tics wouldn't come as often, I noticed, when I was busy concentrating on serving people and moving around.

The van didn't just sell ice creams; it sold all the different makes of fags and crisps and stuff like that, too. I started to enjoy meeting the local punters and taking their orders:

'All right there, John? Two ice-cream cones with raspberry sauce and twenty Lambert & Butler, please, son. Say hi to your mum, will you? How's she keeping? She doing OK?'

It kept me busy, and I liked feeling I was in control of what was happening. I was giving people what they wanted, for once, instead of doing something or saying something no one ever wanted. It gave me a purpose, and I'd not had any purpose in such a long time.

Kevin trusted me. It took a while for me to believe it, but after he'd offered me a job for the whole of the summer holidays, I just had to accept that he did.

A week or two in, he even let me stand outside his special cupboard – the one that no one was allowed in – to keep guard while he mixed up his secret recipe.

I remember standing there, feeling like the most important person in the world, thinking, *This is amazing – look where I am! I wish everyone could see me now.*

I had on these massive health-and-safety gloves, and a hairnet, and I was eating a free strawberry ice cream with wee chunks of real strawberries in it. As I bit through cold, creamy lumps, my chest went all tight – big and full – and it started puffing out through the special blue plastic pinny I had to wear. I felt a bit dizzy, a bit woozy, like the happiness was too much and it might just burst right out of me.

21

On Telly

I left school at sixteen with no qualifications. On a good day, I knew I wasn't stupid, but sometimes it got to me – the thought that folk might think I was.

I'd been stressing about what I'd do next. I didn't feel ready for a proper job. *Who'd take me on, anyway?* So it was a real relief when I got on to a local college course for people with special needs. Did I fit the label? In some ways, aye. It helped not to be picked on any more. In other ways, maybe not. But I didn't care much about that.

What surprised me was how quickly I settled in. The course was about building life skills and getting you ready for work. I took to it straight away – the way it was taught worked for me. It was hands on, and that suited me better.

I made pals with folk who had autism, Down's syndrome, cerebral palsy – and we got on. We had a laugh. I found myself naturally helping them to get around college, or giving them a hand with their work. It felt good being useful. And my confidence started to grow with the routine and sense of purpose that college gave me.

Not long into that first term at college, the chair of the Tourette's Support Group got in touch with Mum to say he'd been contacted by a producer who was working for the BBC. They were making a documentary about Tourette's, he said, and he'd thought of Mum and me straight away. They wanted to see a few people initially, to see who'd work best, so it wasn't a given, he explained, but would we be on for having a chat with them?

Mum said she'd need to talk to me first, but she thought it sounded interesting – maybe even something important to be part of.

I agreed. Anything that helped raise awareness had to be a good thing, I reckoned. And if it meant even one person had an easier time of it than I did, then it was worth it.

'Count me out,' Dad said, without hesitating, when we told him. 'If it happens, then I won't be having anything to do with it. I don't want to be on telly.'

Fair enough. I wasn't massively keen to be on telly either, nor was Mum, but it wasn't about that. As far as I saw it, that was the bit we'd just have to bear to get people to know about Tourette's.

I don't remember being disappointed with Dad. I think I'd suspected from the start that he wouldn't be up for it. My parents' marriage was in real difficulties by now, so I think this just gave him another reason to spend more time out of the house and away from us.

The producer and an assistant came to Galashiels for a week. They visited us every day, spending time with us at home, filming me with Mum going about our day-to-day lives. Once I got past my nerves, I started to quite like having them around. They were lovely, both of them – positive, considerate people, and easy to be with. It was such a novel thing for me to have someone actually take an interest in me, but in a positive, non-threatening way. I couldn't think when I'd last had that. Maybe when I was ten, and getting quite good at football? So it took a while for me to trust it was real, and to settle and relax into it.

A few weeks later we got a call from the production company to say they'd like us to be the focus of the documentary. They'd been looking at five other families, the producer said, and out of all the stories, without question, ours was the most impactful. I felt such a jumbled-up mix of emotions when I heard that: fear and worry about what I was letting myself in for, and excitement – there was no denying the thrill of it, the buzz: *I'm going to be on telly!* But I felt a bit sad about it, too. *Why was my story the most impactful?* Because I had the worst case, out of everyone – that's what it meant.

The film crew started to come up to Galashiels for long weekends soon after. I hadn't been expecting so many of them. I remember watching from the window as all these cars drew up outside, amazed by how many people got out, one after the other. I didn't know anything about TV production – why would I? I think I'd been expecting just a crew of two, like last time. *Why is everyone wearing black? There are so many beanie hats. Is that a London or a TV thing? Or both?*

The producer told us that the documentary was going to be called *John's Not Mad*, and it was being made for the *Q.E.D.* series. I'd heard of *Q.E.D.* This was a big deal, a way bigger deal than I'd realized. Now I had a sense of the scale of it, I realized just what an opportunity this was for me. I had this one chance – a chance in a lifetime, it felt like – to explain myself to a massive audience, and maybe if they saw it on telly, people might actually be understanding and open-minded – *you just never know.*

I always got uptight before the crew arrived. I was a bit jittery and anxious for a while, but as I got to know them all, I started to enjoy having them around more and more.

As I spent time with them, I learnt what all their different roles were. Fascinated, I quizzed the sound guy, the lighting guy, asking how their kit worked, watched the cameraman at work, chatted to the producers and assistants, soaking it all in.

I soon realized that going into town with a film crew in tow was actually a bit of a blessing – I was protected by them being there. It was the first time I'd felt safe out in public since my Tourette's had started. Nobody was going to have a go at me now. I wasn't about to get jumped or punched in the face. Nobody would spit at me, not with all these folk around.

The crew filmed me going about my day – at college, in the supermarket, fishing by the river – and I got used to it. I even liked some of the fuss and attention. I'd always linked attention with trouble, tried to keep my head down most of the time, but this was different. People would crowd round to watch when we were filming, not angry, just curious and excited.

What were we up to? Why were they filming me?

At first someone from the crew would explain, but soon I was answering folk myself.

No one was shouting stuff at me any more, no one yelled 'Spaz!' across the street. Now they were listening, asking questions. I think being filmed made the Tourette's seem more real to them – something to take seriously, not just brush off.

It felt like something was shifting, not just in other people, but in me too. I wasn't so quick to apologize, and I started to feel more sure of how I handled it – and a bit less ashamed.

The production budget was tiny, apparently, which surprised me. I'd thought because it was being made for the BBC it would be big bucks all the way, but no.

There was no money for studio hire, so the crew made a pretend one instead, in one of their hotel bedrooms, sneaking me in there, past reception, whenever they wanted to interview me, with the hotel none the wiser.

They'd hang up a bedsheet behind me to make it look like a proper big studio. You couldn't tell when you'd see it on camera – it just looked dead professional.

It was a wee while after the filming was over, when I got a call from the producer to say that the neurologist with whom they'd filmed an interview for the documentary had asked if he could speak to me. His name was Oliver Sacks.

'He's one of the world's leading experts on Tourette's,' she said.

'Ah, OK,' I said. 'That's why his name sounds familiar.'

'He's also a bestselling author,' she said. 'He's written about Tourette's in his book *The Man Who Mistook His Wife for a Hat*, and he wrote a book called *Awakenings* – you might have heard of him because of that?'

I got myself a bit tied up in knots before the call, fretting about showing myself up to this highfalutin expert – *What if I don't know the answers? What if I tic? What if he uses words I don't even know? What if, what if, what if* . . . And then the phone rang.

Oliver Sacks wasn't in any way what I expected. Thank God. He was funny and relaxed and friendly, the absolute opposite of the intimidating, uptight doctor I'd been imagining.

We blethered away for a while, about this and that, and when we moved on to Tourette's he had this lovely, gentle curiosity about him, which made it really weirdly easy to open up to him.

'I'm interested to know how you're coping with the condition, John,' he said after we'd been talking for a half-hour or so.

'I don't like it,' I said. 'I just wish it would just go away.'

'Of course,' he said. 'Go on. I want to hear more.'

'Sometimes, I don't know how I can just keep on living my life, knowing that I have to deal with this condition for ever,' I said, grateful to be on the phone so he couldn't see I was crying.

'John, you need to listen to me.'

'Aye,' I said, 'I'm listening.'

'First and foremost, this is what you must do.'

I remember hanging there, not blinking, not ticcing, just waiting, thinking, *Tell me, just tell me.*

'You have to find a way to come to terms with this condition,' he said. 'It may sound difficult, it may even sound ludicrous, but you have to accept that there will be elements of life that you may not be able to partake in, and you are going to have to find ways to adapt to that.'

'OK . . .' I said, wanting him to carry on and keep telling me what to do. He sounded so definite and certain.

'Acceptance is very, very important,' he said. 'You need to learn, not just about Tourette's but about *John* with Tourette's. You must accept that *this is me*, and that your life is going to be dominated by this condition. Only then can you be in a position to thrive and get on with your life,' he said. 'Because if you don't accept it . . .'

'Then what?'

'Well, John,' he said, 'it will haunt you for the rest of your days.'

I've been guided by his words ever since.

There was a delay in the documentary being aired. It took ages before it was on TV. The BBC didn't want to have it on before the watershed, they said, because of all the swearing; they wanted it on at eleven p.m. The production company and *Q.E.D.* stood firm. *That defeats the purpose*, they said. *We need families to see it; we're not going to get the audience we need if you do that. We want the whole nation to be able to sit down and watch this.*

It went to court in the end. Thankfully, the judge was on side and agreed with them that it was vital for it to be shown on prime-time TV.

The documentary was given a nine p.m. slot, with the BBC news even being postponed until after it was aired.

In the time that had passed, Dad had left home. We'd all seen it coming, but it was still a shock when Mum announced it to us. Dad wasn't there when Mum told us all. I don't know where he was – probably down the pub again. I've blocked out most of the memory of his going, maybe because it was too painful for me to hang on to.

Day to day, Dad not living with us wasn't a massive change. Because it had happened so slowly, we'd barely noticed that he'd been with us less and less.

It was hard, though, and sad for all of us, even so. There was something about the finality of it, having to face the fact that this was it: we were a single-parent family from now on.

I blamed myself – of course I did. Blaming myself was

my go-to back then. I had to have had something to do with their break-up. I'd heard the rows they'd have about me, so my Tourette's must have, at the very least, contributed to it.

When I couldn't sleep, I'd tell myself it was entirely because of me.

If I wasn't here, if I didn't have it, then they'd still be together.

Maybe not – who knows? Sometimes in life, no matter how hard you want them, no matter how hard you try to think the answers into existence, it makes no difference, does it? You still never get them. Things don't always tie up in the way that you'd like, and you're just left to wonder and wonder.

I felt so protective over Mum, I hated her being alone, even though, bit by bit, she'd been alone for months, maybe even years by now.

I wanted her to be happy. I yearned for it. I felt like Mum being happy would make the whole family happy, spreading out to all of us, like osmosis.

What about the documentary? Its imminent airing began to take on an added weight for me.

I fretted about it all the time. *Will that make things better or worse?*

I wanted Mum to feel proud that we'd done it.

What if she hates it?

I was desperate for her to be happy that we'd made the right decision.

I needed this to be a *good thing* for us, too – maybe here it was at last, something to finally offset all the bad stuff and flip all the crap that had come our way on its head for ever.

I didn't want to watch the documentary with my family.

The thought of seeing it was already overwhelming as it was, and I knew myself well enough by then to know that if I was feeling too many emotions, in the presence of too many people, then I'd be sent into a massive great whirling vortex of anxiety that might take me hours, even days to climb out of.

Mum and my brother and sisters were going to watch it together in the sitting room, and I opted to watch it by myself, in my bedroom, on my little black-and-white portable TV.

It was such a strange sensation, watching myself on television.

Is that me? Is that what I look like? Do I sound like that? Thoughts like that kept getting in the way, distracting me, and I had to keep talking to myself, calming myself down enough to concentrate.

'John! Come up!' Mum was shouting at me the minute the credits rolled.

I remember I was crying with relief as I came up the stairs. I felt like I was floating. I couldn't feel my feet on the stairs – that's how light I was.

Everyone knows now, I kept thinking.

It was like I'd just come out with Tourette's.

'Well? What do you think?' Mum had to keep on asking, because I couldn't speak at first. It was too much. All of it. It was way too big.

Mum was smiling. *She was actually smiling!* There were a couple of bits, of course, but just a couple, she said, that she wished they hadn't put in, but yes, she *thought it was pretty good*, which made me cry even more. If you know my mum, that basically means she thought it was amazing, Oscar-worthy. The best thing ever.

The day after the documentary I was jittery and wired and all over the place. My hands were shaking as I shoved my shoes on in the hallway.

'Where are you off to, John?' Mum was frowning, concerned; she wasn't used to me being in a hurry to get out of the house.

'I want to walk into town.' I'd never thought those words would come out of my mouth.

'What on earth for?' Mum couldn't believe it, either. She'd had to drag me into town for years now.

'I want to see what people's reactions are to the documentary last night,' I said, grabbing my coat. 'I'm desperate to know.'

'OK, well, don't be going too far, OK?' she said, helping me into a sleeve. 'Just go down the high street and come back up. I don't want you hanging around. What if you get beat up or something?'

I wavered then, and I stood there in the hall for about ten minutes, trying to pluck up the courage.

'No. I'm doing it, Mum. I've got to do it,' I said.

'Well, don't expect too much, son,' she called after me as I headed out of the door. 'You just might not get what you hope for. You need to prepare yourself for that, OK?'

That's just how Mum is: always erring on the side of caution, verging on doom and gloom.

I do sometimes wonder where I got my optimism from.

When I got to the high street, I stood for a minute and just looked, as I took a deep breath in. Usually, my presence created a sea change. I'd tic, yell out something, and the steady flow of people would be disrupted in an instant, the current turning as people started crossing the road to avoid me.

Just thinking about the impact I had – the fear and the humiliation – brought on a tic. 'Fuckers, the lot of you!' I shouted, flinching with embarrassment as I waited for the ripple effect.

It didn't happen. Well, it did, just not in the way that it used to. People changed the direction they were walking, but now instead of walking away from me, they were actually coming towards me.

'Hi, John,' a dad with a toddler said. 'I thought you done brilliant on the TV last night. I just wanted to say well done.'

Now Mr Jenkins, who ran the hardware shop, came out to pat me on the back and tell me how proud everyone was of me.

Behind him, a local lad, Pete Williams from my year in school, was standing waiting to talk to me.

'I want to say sorry,' he said with a nervous cough. 'I used to think you should be institutionalized. I don't know why I thought that. I had no idea.'

'It's no bother, honestly,' I said. 'Thank you for saying that, though. It means a lot to me.'

'Any time you want to come and mess with us – you know, me and the gang,' he said, 'just say.'

I wanted to stay and lap it all up, but I kept thinking of Mum hovering, waiting for me at home, so reluctantly I started to head back.

'Hey, John!' A lad I recognized from the year below was waving as he hurried across the road to get to me.

'All right, mate?' he said, grinning. 'I'm Murray.'

'Yeah, I know,' I said. 'I remember you.' Murray was one of those lads that everyone knew. I'd watch him at school sometimes, from the edge of the playground, in awe of the way that everyone liked him, how he'd just flit between groups with nae bother.

'Just to say, I thought you did great last night,' he said. 'I wanted to say, good on you.'

'Cheers for that,' I said, repeating his words in my head, hoping to make them sink in.

'Do you want to come and play football with us?' he said. 'Tomorrow night? Up at the Catholic school?'

'Oh, aye, I know where you mean,' I said, trying to keep it together. 'That could be good, yeah,' I said. 'I'll see' – thinking, *I'm there*. 'If I've not got anything on, I might come and join you,' I said, thinking, *Hell and high water won't stop me*.

'That's great,' Murray said with a thumbs-up. 'See you there, six o'clock.' He was heading back over the zebra crossing now. 'Oh.' He stopped, mid-crossing, and turned back to me. 'And, John, when you come, you dinnae need to worry about what you say. Do you hear me? You can just let it out, man, OK?'

I wanted to punch the air when he said that. I felt like running after him and giving him a massive great big bear hug. Instead, I nodded and muttered, 'Nae problem,' as I started running back home, my head filled with images of me playing football again, wondering where I could find my long-lost football boots, thinking, *Do I still fit them? If not, have I got time to go and buy some more?*

The reviews for the documentary were almost all incredibly positive. However, Ofcom had been in touch to say they'd had a major complaint from Mary Whitehouse, who was appalled by the foul language. Of course she was.

Points of View, a popular consumer-led programme at the time, discussed the feedback they'd had from viewers, and while most were resoundingly positive, a few mentioned how disgusting it was to hear me swearing, with someone advising that I needed a good leathering to sort me out.

College had given me a couple of weeks off after the documentary aired, just to rest and take it all in. I remember getting up every morning to answer the door to the postman, and bringing in bundles and bundles of mail. There was so much of it that it wouldn't fit through the letterbox, so he had to knock for me every time.

I didn't know things like this could happen. I don't know how people even got my address. Most of the letters were from well-wishers; some even sent cheques and gifts. I opened every one of them, reading them over and over.

In the end I was sent well over a thousand letters. The occasional one telling me I needed to pray, the odd one bringing up the exorcism thing and the devil and stuff, but those didn't get to me – they were just tiny mad blips in among the constant stream of goodwill.

Letter after letter, proving to me, and to Mum, that we had absolutely – no doubt about it now – done the right thing.

22

Ku Klux Klan

There's so much that's confusing about my condition. Sometimes I look back at something that happened, a memory that stands out for me, and I don't know what to file it under. Funny? Tragic? Embarrassing? It can often be a jumble of all three.

This is a typical example.

It was not long after the documentary aired, and Mum was off to the hairdresser's.

It was sunny – I remember that, because the washing was out in the garden.

'Don't let Floss out the back, will you now?' Mum called as she headed out the door. 'The rabbit's there, remember?' Her voice always sounded different, I noticed – lighter – when she left the house on her own.

'Right, Mum, don't worry, nae problem,' I called back. 'Nae problem,' I repeated, for extra assurance.

So far, so simple. I only had one straightforward instruction to follow, so I was confident – elated, even – to be left alone, to be entrusted with the house and the pets.

There were always pets when I was growing up. At one point we had three dogs, and there was usually at least one rabbit on the go. I've been nuts about animals ever since I can remember, but as my condition progressed, and I hit my teens, I appreciated more and more the unconditional love a pet can give. I could be as ticcy as anything and it made no odds to them.

Back then, we just had the two pets: Floss, a rescue collie, and Snowy the rabbit. They were lovely, but they made for a stressful combination. Floss had to be kept away from Snowy at all costs.

I knew this.

But still.

I was a constantly curious boy, and impatient, always itching to know stuff and look at stuff and asking 'Why?' all the time, 'What about that? How does that work?'

As soon as Mum left, I kept going to the kitchen window, looking out at the washing blowing in the wind. Was it maybe dry already? Should I go out and check?

I just wanted to help. I always wanted to help. If I brought the washing in, it would balance things out, offset some of the daily upset and turmoil I created, and then Mum would be happy and proud of me.

So my stupid action came from a good place, though I appreciate that, in the carnage that followed, the 'good place' part was easy to overlook completely, especially when dealing with a blood-splattered, dying rabbit in your hallway.

I meant no harm.

I never do.

I wasn't thinking. There are times when I overthink, and times when all rational thoughts seem to vacate my head, and this was one of those times. I went out to check the washing – of course, I couldn't help myself – and the next thing I heard was Floss growling and snarling. When I turned around, my stomach dropped, because she had poor, helpless little Snowy in her mouth.

Panic made me act fast. I grabbed the rabbit and shoved Floss into the kitchen in seconds, then I sat down in the hallway and cradled Snowy in my arms. She was still alive but there were spots of blood all over her lovely, pure white fur. As I stared down at her, feeling her helpless, warm little body in my arms, the enormity of my massive fucking cock-up hit me, and I cried and cried.

Mum told me not to. Mum told me not to, I kept thinking, *and now look, now look what I've gone and done.*

A sudden loud banging on our front door made me jump.

Maybe Mum's psychic, I told myself, *maybe she's run back early from the hairdresser's because she sensed it, she knows what her stupid son has just done?*

In the shock of it all, that seemed a perfectly reasonable assumption.

I got to my feet, Snowy still in my arms, and went to open the door, but before I could get to it, a piece of metal darted through the letterbox.

What the fuck's that? I thought as I struggled to open the door, grappling with Snowy and the doorknob.

It wasn't Mum.

It was a man in a white robe, with a white pointy hood, and he was holding a metal crucifix.

I thought of Hammer horror films, the Ku Klux Klan, my mind whirring into overdrive as it tried, and failed, to make sense of what I was seeing.

'Are you John Davidson?' the man asked.

'Aye, that's me,' I said, squinting up at him – the sunshine and all his white get-up made for a blinding combination. 'What are you wanting?'

There were two other men standing behind him, but they were dressed normally, in jeans and T-shirts, which somehow made him look weirder than ever, standing there in the middle of our terraced street.

They seemed to look a bit scared of me, and I thought, *Why are you looking like that? You came here to see me; I'm the one who should be scared*, as I shifted my sticky hands under Snowy and felt the dull plop of blood on my trainer.

'I'm a rabbit killer!' I shouted out, and the man took a step away from me, jerking his head back like I was going to hit him.

'Sorry,' I said. 'Just a tic.'

All three of them started talking, from a safe distance now, but so quickly I couldn't make out a word they were saying. It was like they were speaking in tongues.

The man was holding the cross out in front of me, and he began flicking water on to me.

'What are you doing?' I said, holding up an arm to shield myself. My whole hand was covered in blood.

'We're here to exorcize you,' the man said – kindly slowing down his words for that bit – 'you're possessed by demons.' His voice was deep and bellowing, like a cow. 'And we need to dispel them!' he yelled.

There were curtains twitching now. Brenda, three doors down, was poking her head out of her window.

'Look,' I said, annoyed more than anything, 'I've got to sort my rabbit out. Will you just fuck off?' And I slammed the door shut in their faces.

Blood was everywhere – smeared on the door, all over my

face as I caught my reflection in the hallway mirror – and Snowy looked more like Pinky now.

I called the hairdresser's, which was only two streets away, and asked if I could speak to my mum.

Mum was there in minutes, looking lethal as she marched down the street, with all the foils in her hair, a magazine still in her hand.

You don't mess with Mum. Nobody messes with Mum.

All three of the men visibly shrank at the sight of her, which you would. Anyone would.

'What's your business?' Mum said, waving her rolled-up magazine at them. Even with her foils in, she was an intimidating presence, with her powerful build and immaculate clothing, all neat and put together, her blouse pressed to within an inch of its life.

'We're trying to help you. Your son is possessed,' the hooded man said, but a lot less loudly this time.

'You'll be possessed of a black eye if you don't skedaddle right now,' my mum shouted, setting on them with her magazine.

The neighbours were out of their houses now, taking in the show – these big men cowering behind their held-up hands as the blows rained down, until they muttered an apology and scuttled off down the street, to everyone's cheers and shouts of 'Good riddance!' from Mum.

I was too relieved to be embarrassed, just happy that it was her, and not me, who was the focus of attention for once.

23

Meeting Dottie

After Dad left, things at home got much harder. Home had been difficult for as long as I could remember, but I'd found ways to tolerate it, just about. Not any more.

Mum was *not in a good way*. I heard her state of mind being summed up, in this vague, euphemistic way, by my maternal grandparents, who dropped their voices when I came into the kitchen and changed the subject immediately.

It's because of me.

'Fucking twats!' I shouted. I'd been swearing for so long, but I still made them flinch.

It's OK, I told them in my head. *Don't worry. I know it's all my fault.*

'Not being in a good way' is a bit of a catch-all phrase, isn't it? With Mum, it meant that she had nothing left to give. And I mean nothing. All her reserves were gone. Even before the Tourette's she had been more highly strung than most, but now she was 'a bag of nerves', as they'd say back then. She'd flip out over anything – the smallest thing – and of course my tics were something that anyone would struggle to live with, so now I'd infuriate and upset her in a way that felt cruel to me. I felt guilty just being in the same room as her, knowing any minute now I'd set off a reaction in her that she couldn't seem to come back down from. I'd ruin her evening. Not just her evening; it felt like I was ruining her life.

I couldn't stand the effect I was having on her and my brother and sisters, too, and I blamed myself for all of it.

Dad left us because of me. I kept saying that to Mum, believing it mainly, but still not quite wanting to, holding out for some kind of reassurance from her – *don't worry, son, of course that's not true* – but she was so tired, so 'not in a good way', that all she could do was weakly shake her head, which just confirmed what I already knew. *It was me that had broken my family.*

I spent more and more time out of the house. What else could I do? It was easier for everyone that way.

I went fishing on my own, but when I'd feel like a bit of company, then I'd go and hang out with Murray. He'd become my mate now, and I'd got to know his friends through playing football, and they were a lovely bunch of lads. Murray was younger than me – I was sixteen then, he was fifteen – but he was old for his age; everyone said that about him.

He wasn't as much into football as I was, but we shared a love of dirt bikes. Sometimes, at the weekends, we'd head off to the woods to ride our bikes around the tracks. He was the only one brave enough to take a backie from me, gripping on like mad when a tic would make me suddenly jerk the bike hard to one side.

He wasn't easily scared by things, which had to be a reason he was friends with me.

'Will you come back to ours for tea?' Murray said as we came to his road after an afternoon in the woods.

'*Fuck, no!*' That was a tic, but I meant what I said.

I couldn't think of anything worse.

Whenever we'd say goodbye after hanging out, I think Murray could tell I didn't want to go home. I never told him, but I didn't need to; he always just picked up what I was thinking. I'd known this invite was coming for a while, and I'd been dreading how to say no without seeming rude.

'Sorry, mate, but nah, you're all right,' I said. 'I got to get back.'

'Yeah, right,' he laughed. 'Bet you can't wait.'

Murray's mum, Dottie, was dying of liver cancer. She had maybe six months left to live. I'd wanted to cry when Murray had told me this. He had a younger brother and sister, and a stepdad, Chris, who made his mum happier than she'd been in years, he told me, and they'd only been married six months. I felt so bad for them all. Not that it mattered. I knew if I went in his house, it would be the last thing I'd convey, because a more tic-inducing scenario was hard to imagine.

'Will you just come, though, mate? You dinnae need to fear about Dottie,' Murray said – he never called her Mum – 'she's dead laid-back. You cannae offend her, I tell you.'

We were standing outside his house now, and I could see Dottie looking out the window at us, smiling, waving at us to come in.

There was no time for me to skedaddle. The front door was opening already, and there was Dottie, in the doorway in a wheelchair. She was blonde, and beaming like the sun, with the kindest, nicest face I'd ever seen. *How can she look so happy when she's dying?* I thought. *What is wrong with her?*

'I've brought someone home for tea, Dottie. This is my pal John,' Murray said, turning back to me with a smile and a wink to say, *Sorry, mate, no going back now.*

'Come on in, John,' Dottie said, reversing her wheelchair to let me through. 'You're very welcome.'

'Ha, ha! You're gannae fucking die!' I shouted.

Dottie just looked up at me as I stared back at her, frozen, thinking, *Shoot me, kill me now.*

'Well, that's a change.' She was actually smiling. 'No one knows what to say to me since my diagnosis.' She laughed. 'So thank you – that's the most honest anyone's been to me.'

I didn't know how to take her reaction. It was so far away from what I'd expected, I just stood there looking gormless, I think, until she patted my leg and told me to hurry up and get in so she could shut the door.

Years later, Dottie told me I spent a lot of those early days with them looking completely bewildered, and she was right. I was bewildered by everything. Their house was so different, for one thing, more arty than mine: full of things she'd made, paintings and clay figures, and crocheted blankets all over the place, and there was a piano in the sitting room. I knew Chris was musical; Murray had told me he was writing an opera. I didn't know what to make of that – it intimidated me, I guess. We didn't even listen to music in our house, so the thought of someone making it, too, was more than my head could take.

Chris appeared from the kitchen and greeted me with a friendly smile. Like Dottie, he smiled with his eyes as well as his mouth.

'Ah, I recognize you!' he said. It took me a moment to clock his features, his dark, wavy hair, his round glasses, and for the penny to drop with a great big clunk into my gut.

Yes, we'd met, just last week, when I'd forced a reluctant

Murray to have a kick-about with me on the green outside the community college. Chris was the man who was going into the college – Dottie was working there at the time, I found out later, and he was going in to see her – when I kicked the ball too hard, and it just missed him.

'Can you kick us the ball back, please?' I yelled, ticcing, 'You speccy cunt!'

He didn't shout at me. I'd got so used to being shouted at that it threw me – the calm, confident way he responded. He just stopped and gave me a long, steady look, then said, 'I think you should get your own ball back, don't you?' before walking into the college.

Murray had never let on that he was his stepdad. He knew better than that; it would have only spun me out and set me off ticcing like crazy.

It's a funny one, isn't it? Eating with another family you don't know. I didn't know what to make of any of them at first. They kept laughing at stuff, and singing, and teasing each other, and I just kept thinking about my family and wondering, *Which way is right? Are you meant to laugh all the time like this, or not at all, like we do?*

They wanted to play a card game after we'd eaten, all together, as a family. We didn't have cards at my house, so it felt weird to me, that first time, and I kept shouting out the cards I had, but no one seemed to mind.

'Stop apologizing,' Dottie said. 'We all know you can't help it.'

I wanted to do the washing-up, and no one believed me when I said I liked doing it. I need to keep busy, I said, that's the best way – it still is – to keep the tics at bay.

Left: With my grandmother, 1972.

Below: Me aged four.

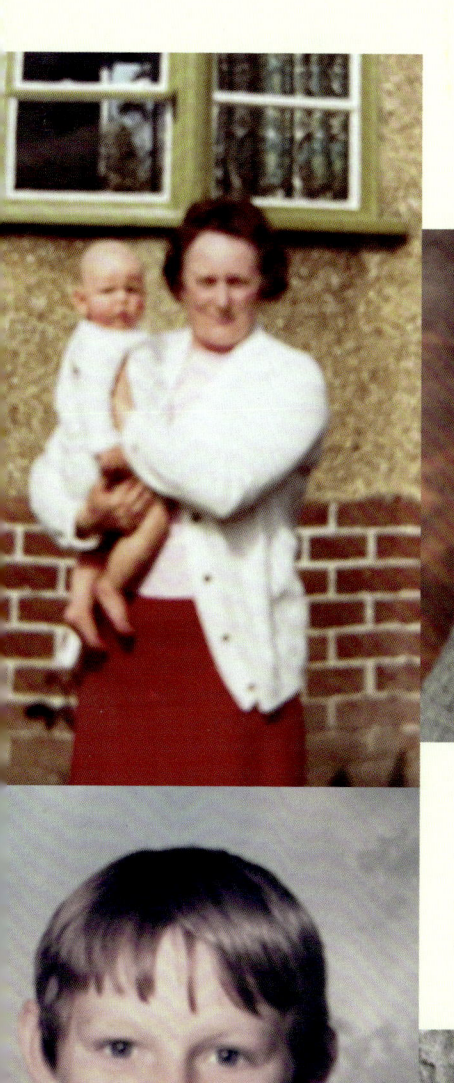

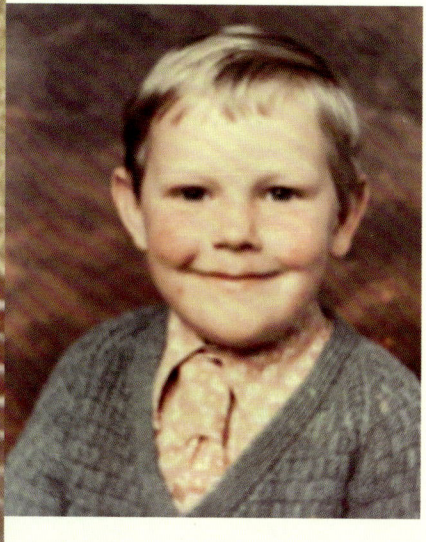

Left: In my secondary school uniform, aged twelve.

Below: The DVD cover of the documentary made when I was sixteen.

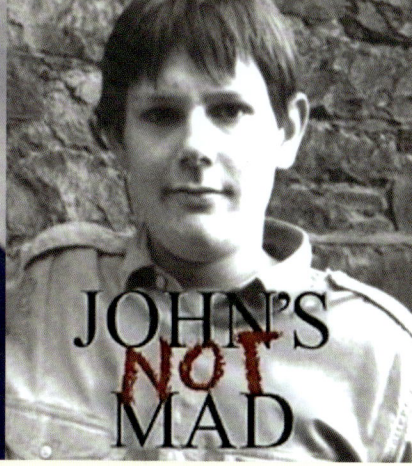

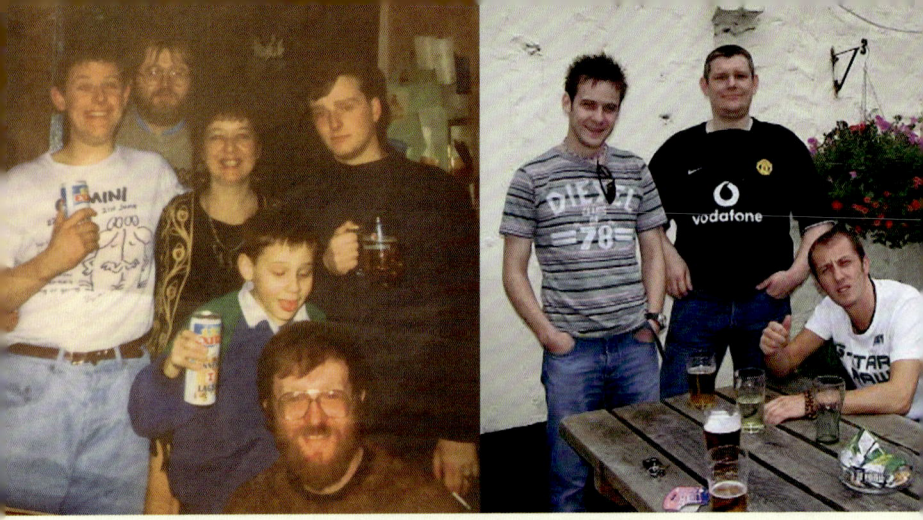

Above left: An early moment with the Achenbach family. (From left to right): me, Dawn's boyfriend Mike, Dottie, Roddy and Andrew, with Chris in the foreground.

Above right: With Roddy and Murray.

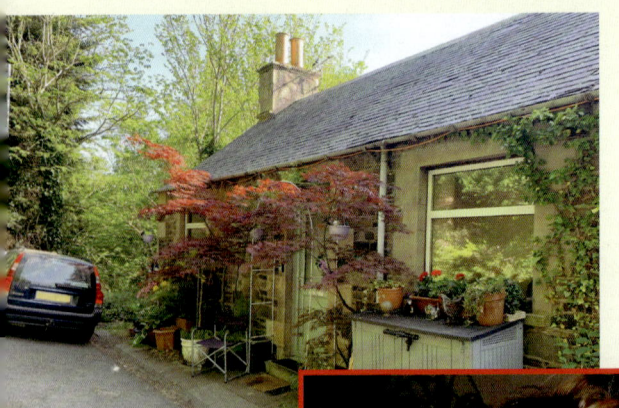

Left: The Achenbachs' home.

Right: With Dottie, 2017.

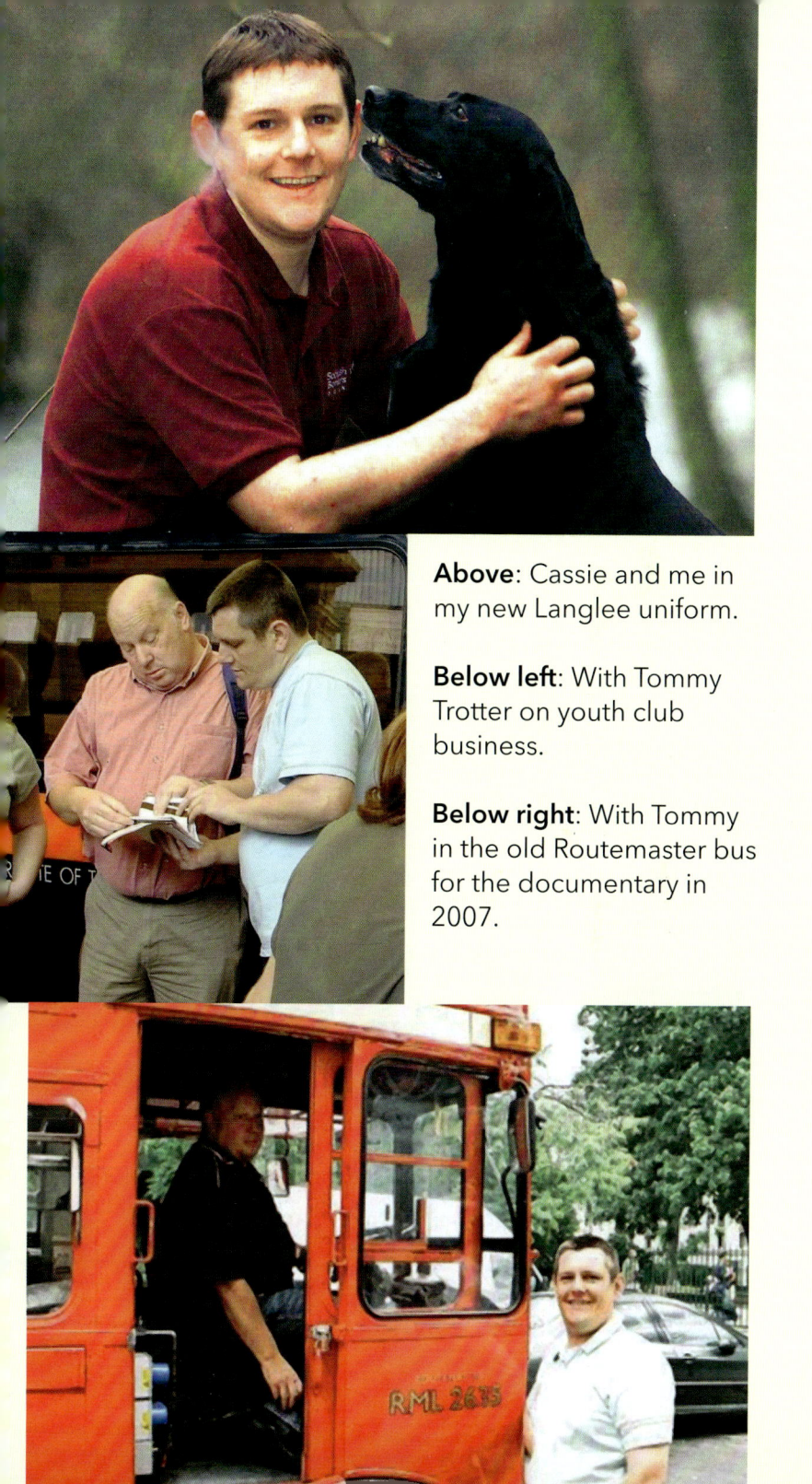

Above: Cassie and me in my new Langlee uniform.

Below left: With Tommy Trotter on youth club business.

Below right: With Tommy in the old Routemaster bus for the documentary in 2007.

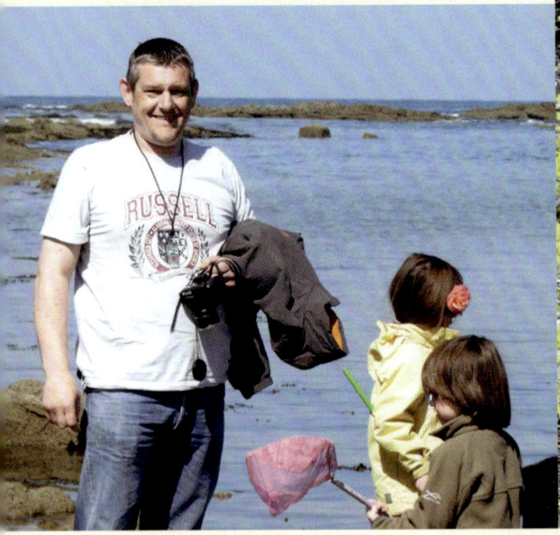

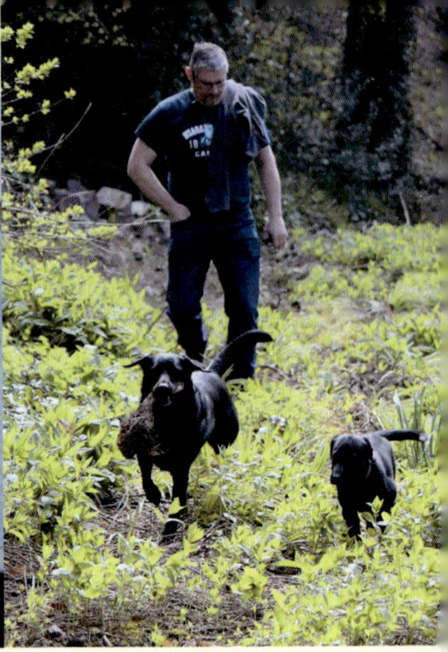

Above left: On holiday in Arisaig.

Above right: Walking the dogs – Tilly is on the left.

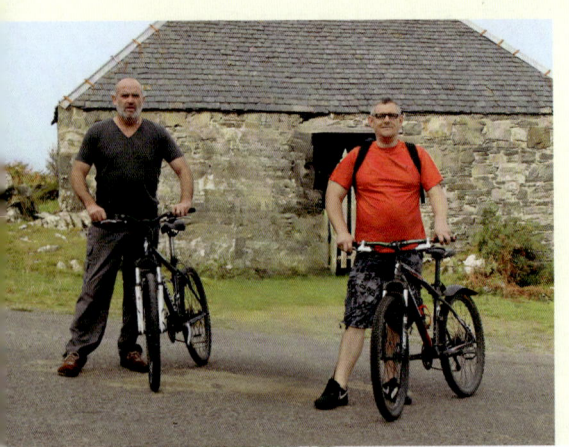

Left: On a cycling holiday with Paul.

Below: Paul and me in Fort William, during the making of a Tourette's awareness video.

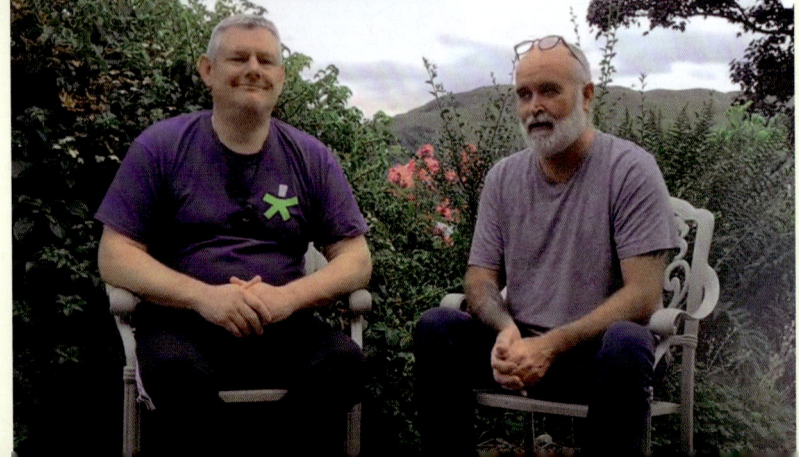

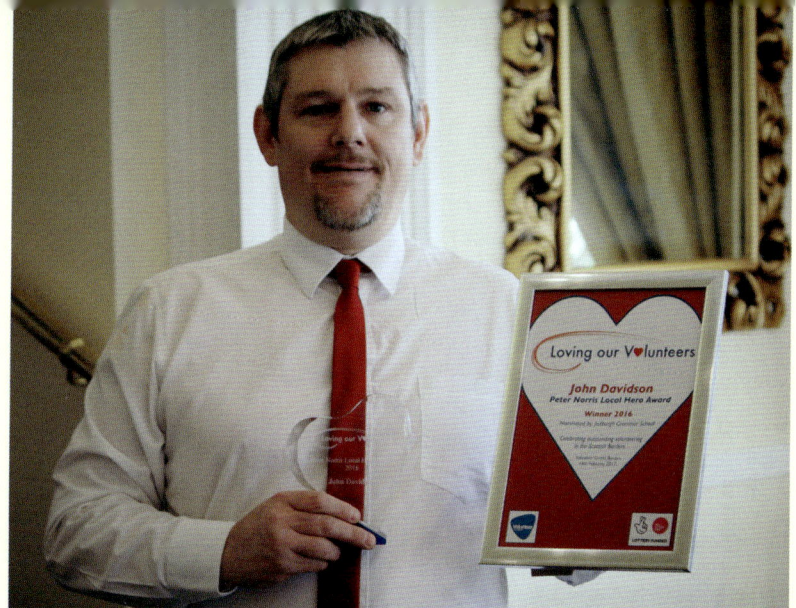

Above: Me with my Peter Norris Local Hero Award for volunteering in the community, 2016.

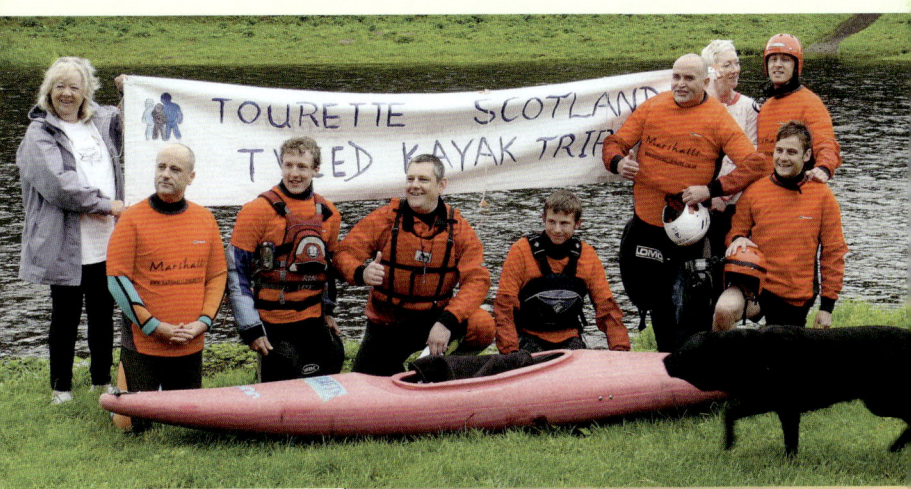

Above: Our 2010 fundraiser for Tourette Scotland – we kayaked eighty miles down the River Tweed.

Right: Tourette action poster.

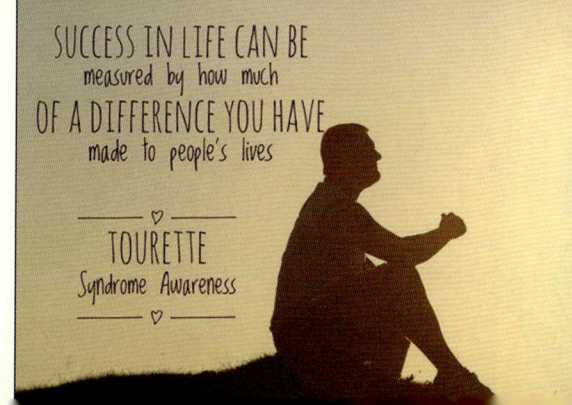

SUCCESS IN LIFE CAN BE *measured by how much* OF A DIFFERENCE YOU HAVE *made to people's lives*

♡

TOURETTE *Syndrome Awareness*

♡

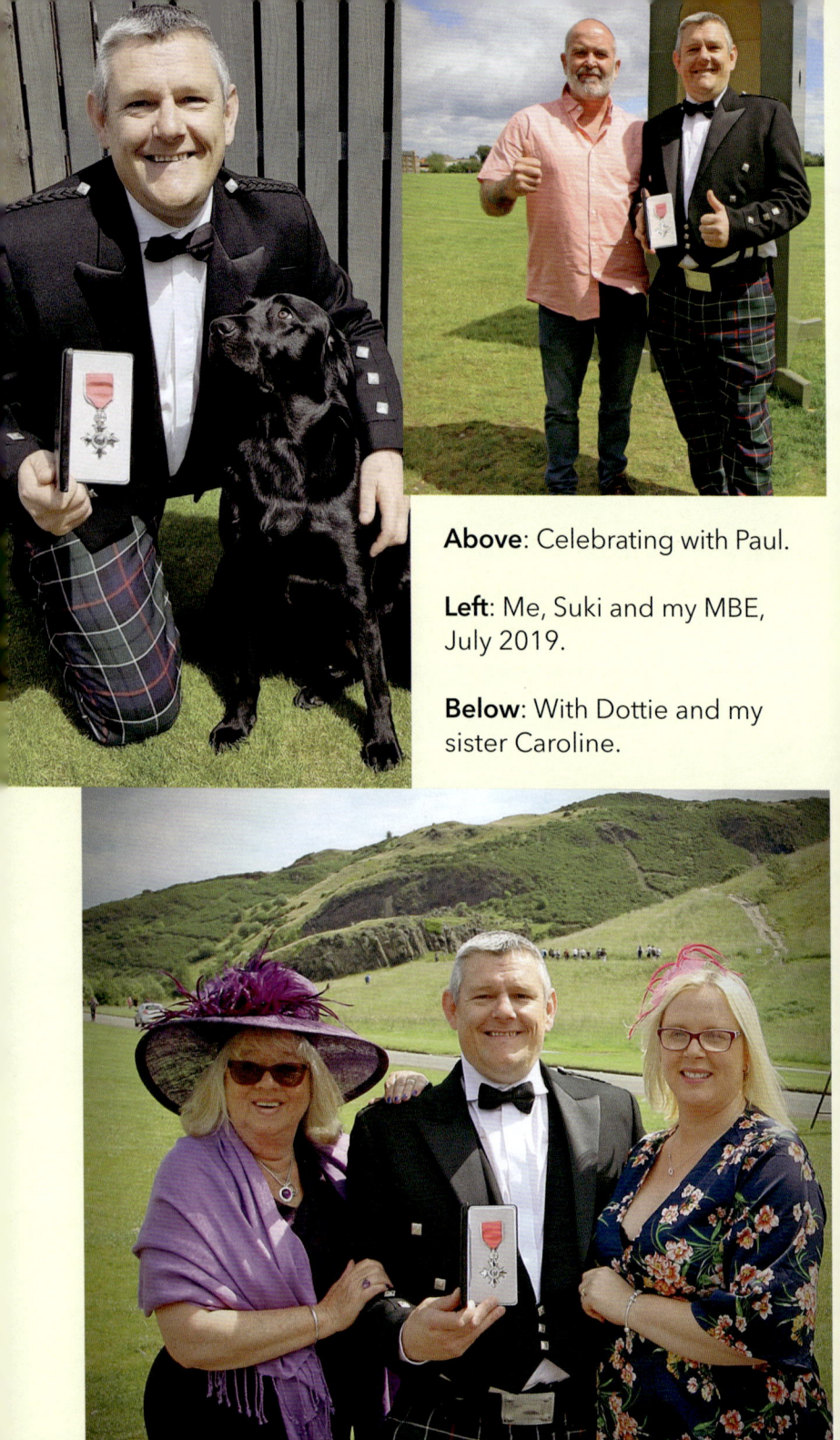

Above: Celebrating with Paul.

Left: Me, Suki and my MBE, July 2019.

Below: With Dottie and my sister Caroline.

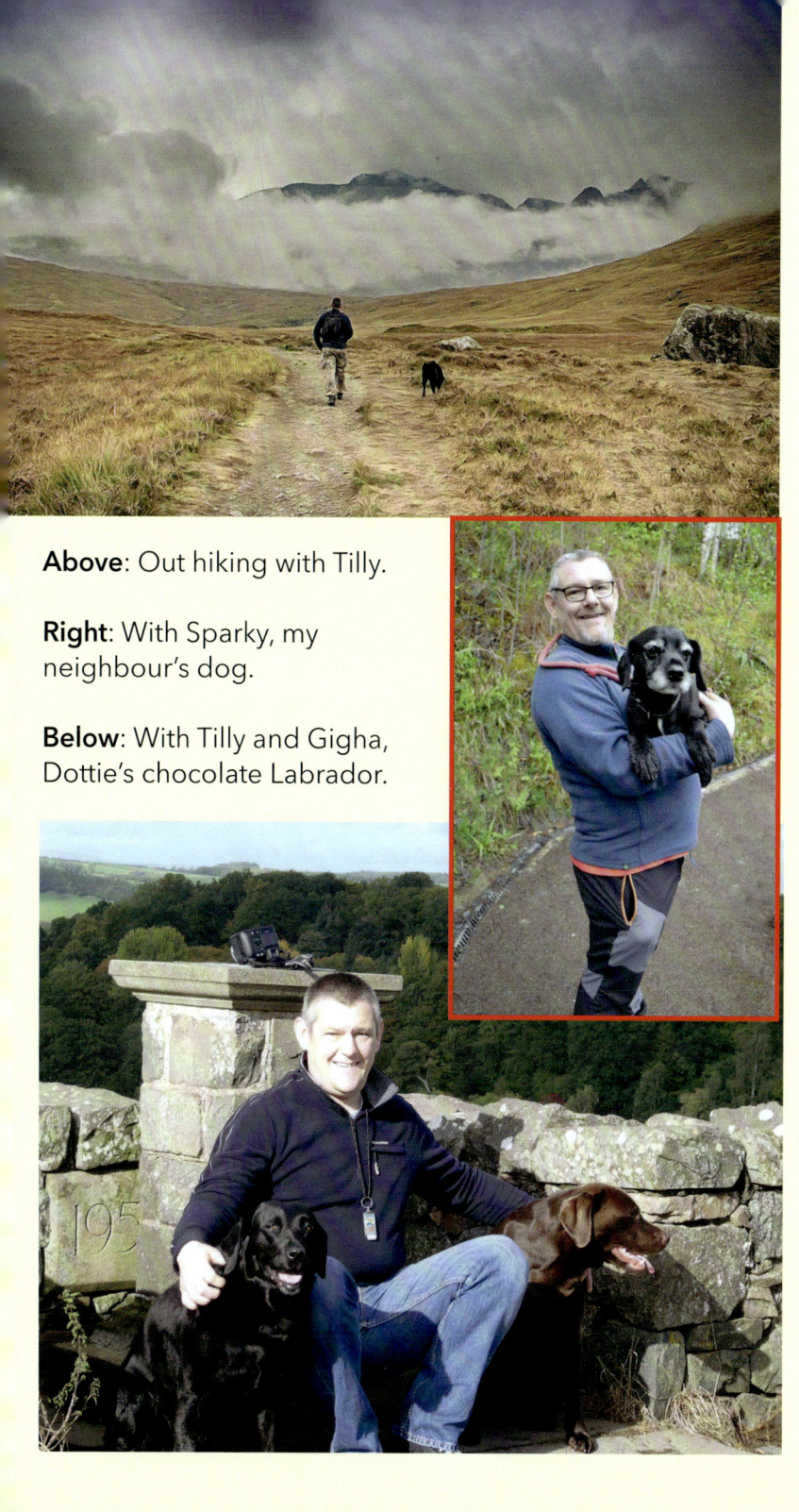

Above: Out hiking with Tilly.

Right: With Sparky, my neighbour's dog.

Below: With Tilly and Gigha, Dottie's chocolate Labrador.

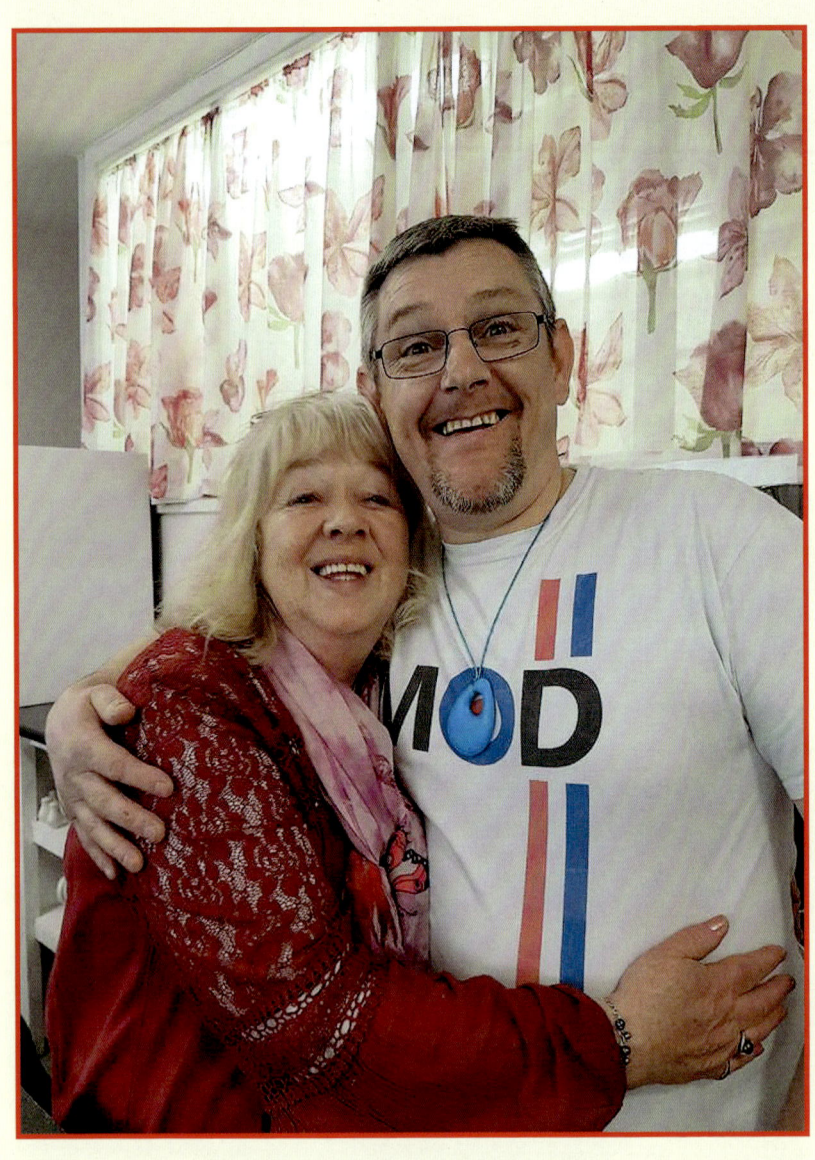

Dottie and me.

'Ah well, never mind, John,' Dottie said, smiling, when I broke a plate by smashing it down in the sink. 'Don't you worry. I'll get us some melamine ones for next time.'

Next time. They were the nicest, happiest-making words I'd heard in such a long time.

24

Moving In

Melamine isn't unbreakable, as it turns out. I was going over to Dottie and Chris's house all the time now, and I kept breaking the new plates Dottie bought for me. I'd smash glasses too, ornaments, vases of flowers, you name it – every time I was over, there'd be something.

Murray said they had a running joke in their family that if a bloody great bull came to their door, Dottie would bring it in and feed it some hay.

Now look! She had me, the proverbial bull in the china shop, wreaking havoc all over the place.

I'd sweat with the shame of it – *sorry about that, sorry, Dottie, I'll buy you another one* – but she never seemed bothered like I was. None of them were – *no worries, it does nae matter, I never liked it anyway.* I knew she was being kind; of course she hadn't filled her house with stuff she didn't like. It made me feel terrible, but the guilt wasn't enough to make me stop going. The pull to be with them was so strong it felt like I had no choice but to be there. It was like a primal, survival thing. I'd been holding my breath for so long, and when I was with them, I could finally let it all out again.

*

After a while I wasn't just going to Murray's house to see him; I wanted to be there no matter what. I started going over there after college. *Dottie could do with another pair of hands; I'll pop over and see if she needs some help* – that's how I justified it to myself, but it wasn't just that. I needed her even more.

For someone who had months to live, Dottie was the most upbeat, positive person I'd ever met – and have ever met since – and it was catching: her glass-half-full way of looking at things. The more time I spent with her, the less empty my glass was. I'd been so used to just putting one foot in front of the other, and now I was busy with Dottie, helping her make her garden look nice for the spring, planting bulbs – *you never know, just in case I'm around to see them come out.*

'Don't bother! You'll be dead soon, you silly twat!' I shouted.

She howled with laughter. 'Aye, but what else can I do, John? I've got to embrace a bit of hope, haven't I?' she said. 'I've got three kids and a brand-new husband. It would be nice to think I gave it my best shot to stick around for them.'

She committed herself to looking on the bright side so fully, wheeling herself off to her room to do a bit of meditating, or reiki, or positive affirmations – something spiritual like that. *All her hippy shit*, as her kids like to say.

That 'making the best out of things' mentality was so new to me. I don't think it had occurred to me until then that I could actually be enjoying myself from time to time. We'd sit side by side, the two of us, and make things together out of clay. She encouraged me to draw and paint with her, and have a go at watercolours. I loved losing myself, just getting into it, and forgetting for a while to be stressed. I didn't think I had much creative talent, but Dottie encouraged me all the way.

'What can I say, John? You've done it again,' she'd say when I showed another of my offerings to her. 'I can really see what you were getting at there.'

'Can you?' I'd say, squinting at it, because it looked like a right mess to me.

'Oh, aye.' She'd be nodding and smiling. 'Lovely use of colour you've got there. Keep going, keep up the good work.' And I liked to think I was pleasing her, so I would.

I don't blame my family – it wasn't intentional – but I think the message I'd got from them was that life – and my life in particular – was to be tolerated, and my condition was something I'd have to bear, rather than work with. *Keep taking the meds.* I hated what the meds did to me, but I took them all the same, knowing that it made things easier for everyone at home if I was blunted – barely conscious at times – which had to be better, *anything* had to be better, than causing a scene.

'Does your mum mind that you come over here all the time?'

I was pushing Dottie in her wheelchair one morning, taking her to the post office to get her family allowance. It was a steep hill down into town, and I could feel a tic building: the urge to let go of the handles.

'It's nae bother to her,' I said, sweating now with the effort of holding on to her.

Don't let go. For fuck's sake, John, concentrate. 'She's fine with it,' I said, which was easier than telling her that Mum didn't know, because, yes, of course, it would have been a massive bother to her. What mum would be OK with that?

Their son finding another family? Not mine. But Mum never asked what I was up to, and I didn't tell. I think it suited us both fine that way, having that bit of space we needed from each other.

'OK, darlin', well, as long as you're sure about that?' Dottie said as we reached the main road, turning back to look at me, eyes narrowed. Just checking, I think, giving me a chance to confess.

'We love you being with us – you know that, don't you? But I would nae want her to be upset about it, that's all,' she said, letting out a shriek as I shoved her forward into the path of an oncoming bus.

'No, Dottie, sorry!' I shouted, pulling her out of the way just in time, yanking the wheelchair back on to the pavement as the bus sped past, horn blaring.

She couldn't stop laughing. I couldn't believe it. People were walking past, tutting and glaring at us, but Dottie didn't care. It just made her laugh all the more.

'Are you no mad with me?'

She was shaking her head, catching her breath.

'Nothing scares me any more, John,' she said. 'Besides, that would be an easier, quicker way to go than the way they told me I'd be going. There are worse ways to go than being hit by a bus.'

My arms were still shaking by the time we got to the queue at the post office. I had to have a cigarette to calm myself down.

'I can see you're still stressing, John, but honestly you don't need to be.' Dottie turned back to pat my hand. 'I trust you. I know you'd never actually do it.'

I didn't know if she was right or not.

I'd never had anyone use the word 'trust' before in relation to anything to do with me.

I'd give it a go. I'd try to sit at the table to eat with everyone when I was at Dottie and Chris's, but my food-spitting tic made it hard sometimes. No one pretended to like it, but they all took it pretty well considering, ignoring it as much as they could. Dottie just gave everyone napkins, so they could all shield their faces from the oncoming mouthful, but they really had to be quick off the mark.

When my spitting got out of hand, I'd go and sit in the lounge, facing the fireplace, like I did back at home. I didn't mind doing it at Dottie's, though – it felt more like a practical solution than a shameful thing. Perhaps because I'd chosen to and hadn't been ordered to because Mum said I was too disgusting to eat with.

The more time I spent at Dottie and Chris's, the harder it was to go home. I hated getting back to mine after tea and knowing that I was disturbing the peace. I think that the longer I wasn't there, the more my family realized just how disruptive I was, and the less tolerant they became of me. I'm not criticizing them. I would have been the same, I'm sure, but it meant that I felt increasingly ostracized by my own family. The house had to be a lot calmer without me in it, and so no one could pretend to be happy to see me. Teenage siblings don't tend to be polite to each other, do they?

I used to quite enjoy the way that me and my brother and sisters would rip into each other. I think I liked the back-and-forth of it, the way it made me feel an integral part of things. But now I'd come home to be greeted by everyone groaning at the sight of me, which had quite the opposite effect.

I told Dottie my mum was going away for the weekend. She wasn't going anywhere – she never did – but desperate measures were required. I knew Dottie wouldn't want to think of me home alone without my mum; her heart was way too wide open for that.

I'm not sure she believed me when I told her; she gave me one of her 'are you sure about that now?' looks. I've never been that good at lying, even before the Tourette's, but she invited me to stay the night all the same.

I pretty much moved in from that day.

Dottie likes to say she invited me in for tea and I ended up staying for twenty-five years, and she's not far wrong about that.

We never made it official. It had been happening already, I guess, bit by bit; I'd been gradually becoming a part of their family for months. Maybe we didn't even fully notice it. There was a natural ease to it – somehow it just made a strange kind of sense.

There was no other way. That's what it felt like – to me, at least. Dottie and Chris must have had chats about it, I'm sure, wondered what exactly they were taking on and the impact it would have on all of them, but if they had any concerns, they hid them well from me, and they never made me feel anything but welcome.

I look back now, and I'm astonished by their kindness and generosity. I think it's such a natural part of the way the whole family is – they just made it seem so normal, *no big deal*. Sometimes you have to stand back from things, don't you? To fully see and appreciate something. I still can't believe that I found them.

Not long after I first stayed the night, I was given my own

room. I'm guessing my night-time tics on the sitting-room sofa were keeping everyone up. I could have Roddy's room, Dottie said – the box room – and Roddy could move in with Dawn. *Is this going to be OK?* It worried me. I worried about everything. I didn't want to put anyone out; I never wanted to piss anyone off. Roddy was up for it, though. His room was so tiny, and Dawn had always had the biggest bedroom by miles, he said, and she had bunk beds and that had never been fair. He'd always wanted to be in a bunk bed. He was still at that easy-to-please age when bunks were seen as the ultimate: peak bed.

Not long after I moved in, when I was seventeen, Dottie and Chris said they'd found me someone to see in Edinburgh, some eminent psychotherapist with a special interest in Tourette's. I was keen to talk to him, but the thought of the journey there made me anxious. Edinburgh was a long bus ride away and I hated being in confined spaces with strangers.

I asked Murray to come with me, and he was up for it – he was always up for stuff. 'We'll make a day of it,' he said, 'do a bit of shopping.' He was into his clothes and that was rubbing off on me, and for the first time since my Tourette's had come on, I'd started to take an interest in how I looked again. I bought myself a new pair of boots especially for our trip to the city: lace-up leather ones like the Caterpillar boots that everyone was into back then. I remember checking myself out in the mirror before we left and thinking I looked quite the business.

We talked all the way up on the bus, and I ticced a bit, but nothing like I could have done, because Murray has always been brilliant at distracting me. He knows just to keep me talking. When my mind's occupied it's like there's less room for the tics to find a way in. Sometimes I shouted out the odd 'Fuck!' and a passenger would mutter their disapproval, but Murray gave them his 'do you have a problem?' look and that usually shut them up. I think it was his nice, open face, and the fact that he dressed well and had this easy, relaxed confidence about him: it all gave him an unusual amount of gravitas for a fifteen-year-old kid. Murray could get people to listen. I envied him that, but didn't begrudge him for it. It meant I always felt so much safer when he was with me.

I had my session with the psychotherapist, who said things like, 'Hmm, I see,' and, 'I understand,' and, 'But how does that make you feel?'

It felt odd to me at first, someone I didn't know asking me all these questions – being a wee bit nosy, it felt like – but after a while I got into it.

I said yes, I'd like to see him again, fighting back the niggling disappointment I had in the back of my mind, because while maybe he might help me to feel a wee bit better about things, he wasn't going to do what I wanted – he wasn't going to fix my Tourette's.

The day went downhill after my session. Edinburgh was quite rough back then, and it set me on edge and my tics started ramping up. Murray was having to deploy his diplomacy skills non-stop, stepping in between me and the offended person, left, right and centre. 'Aye, no worries now, he nae means it, he's all right.'

I couldn't wait to get back on the bus, and nor could Murray. The bus was busier than it had been on the way up, which made me tense and wound up.

I hate the feel of being surrounded by strangers, and I could feel my heart speeding up as we sat down at the back, sweat breaking out on my forehead. Everyone was looking, and I couldn't stand it. I get this very specific dull, sick kind of feeling, like giving in to the inevitability of what follows next, because that all-eyes-on-me scenario is guaranteed, always, to bring out a reaction in me.

'OH, FUCK!' I yelled it really loudly – even for me, because Murray's hands went straight over his ears and he was used to my yelling.

I could see the driver puffing up, and now he was getting up in that deliberately slow way from the driver's seat. 'You all right?' he said, turning to face us, and it wasn't in a caring, sharing kind of way. The question was very much rhetorical.

I could see a vein twitching on his neck. He had the thickest neck I'd ever seen, and the look of someone who took steroids: muscles and veins all over the place. Bricks and shithouses sprang to mind.

'FUCKING HELL!'

'Now you're just taking the piss,' the driver said. 'Get off my bus!'

'Whoa!' Murray stepped forward. 'You don't understand – he's got Tourette's. It's involuntary; he can't help it.'

'I don't fucking care what he's got. You can get the fuck off my bus!' Flecks of spit came out of the driver's mouth as he shouted.

'So it's all right for you to swear at us, is it?' Murray said. He's never been scared of anyone.

Meanwhile I was just standing there, sweating with shame, my feet all hot and swollen in my brand-new Caterpillar-style boots.

'You're going to kick us off, then, are you? In the middle of

Edinburgh?' Murray said. 'We've got no money. We've spent all our money on the bus.'

'I don't care!' You could really tell he meant that. 'Get off my bus!'

None of the passengers did anything; no one interjected to help us.

So that was that. We had no choice but to go.

There were no mobile phones back then, and we walked miles in search of a payphone, both of us crying on and off all the way. My tics made me shove my feet into the tarmac as I walked, so soon the sole was coming off one of my pride-and-joy boots. Murray had to find some string and tie it round my foot so we could carry on with the search, my loose sole making a *slap, slap* sound on the pavement.

When at last we found a working payphone, Murray called Dottie and tearfully explained where we were.

I could hear her outraged voice, all high with indignation, buzzing through the receiver. 'Aye, aye.' Murray had to hold the receiver away to protect his hearing. 'OK then, yeah, Dottie, no worries, will do.'

We were to wait there, Dottie said, *promise not to wander off.*

Before long, an empty bus arrived to pick us up, and it took us all the way back to Galashiels, just the two of us.

You don't mess with Dottie, or anyone who knows her. If you're aware of that from the start, it can save you a lot of bother in the long run.

I was in full-on teenage-boy mode now, which meant my tics became a bit one-track for a while.

'I'm having a wank!' was a regular one I'd shout out, though sometimes my tics would be more obscure. 'Jellyfish sex!' came from nowhere and stuck around for a bit.

'I've got a gay leg!' I first shouted that one out when we were playing cards together.

'Oh yeah?' Murray said, looking at me over his cards. 'Which one is it, then? Left or right?'

At Dottie's it never mattered what I said, but it made being out in public more stressful than ever for me.

I had a phase of shouting, 'I'm a homosexual!' Sometimes, though, I could catch it halfway through and change it to 'I'm a home . . . owner!' and that took on a life of its own. 'I'm a homeowner!' I'd yell, over and over, and that became a common tic for a while, too.

Years later, when I came over to Dottie's, all excited, beers in hand, to celebrate because I'd bought my council house, Murray came into the kitchen, grinning from ear to ear.

'Is it true, pal?' he said, giving me a massive hug. 'Finally, mate! You can say it!'

'I don't get you,' I said, handing him a beer.

'You're a *homeowner*!' he said.

Everyone cracked up, and though sometimes it was hard for me to laugh at my tics, this time I couldn't help but join in. Murray was always taking the piss – funny was the norm with him – but I remember him being especially dead pleased with himself for that one.

I really wanted a girlfriend. Murray had a girlfriend now, and she'd come back to Dottie's, and they'd disappear off to his room together. I have to admit, I felt a bit jealous, and that would stress me out and make me tic.

'Murray's having it off!'

Dottie was hard to wind up, but it would always get to her when I did that.

'Stop telling tales, Davidson!' She'd taken to calling me by my surname lately, which was the opposite of formal coming from Dottie – a term of endearment, and I loved it.

'But it's *true!*' I said.

'I don't care if it is. Try and respect their privacy, will you?'

But privacy wasn't something I could give anyone easily, and Dottie's disapproval – even the word 'privacy' – would trigger me and make me need to tic all the more.

Murray knew I was feeling left behind, and he wanted to help me out. He was always kind like that.

'You just need to practise chatting to lasses,' he said, so he brought a couple of his mates back to Dottie's one afternoon.

I was more relaxed at Dottie's than at college, and when I could see the lasses had a genuine curiosity about the Tourette's, I found myself explaining what it was like for me.

'Something just pops into my head,' I said. 'It's not even what I'm necessarily thinking, but it just comes out.'

'But can you no think of something nice?' the taller of the two said. She had massive flicks in her hair, just like Sharon from *Grange Hill*, and I tried not to let that intimidate me.

'What do you mean?' I said. 'Give me an example.'

'Well, the things you come out with are, like, swearing, or spitting,' she said. 'Can you no just make the thoughts nice ones? About puppies? Or flowers? Stuff like that?'

I could feel a tic building. *Flowers, flowers*, I was thinking. *Make it nice.*

'*Fucking poppies up your arse!*'

'Oh,' she said. I remember the look of dismay on her face, which set me off again.

'*You pansy bastards!*'

They didn't stay too long after that.

25

Dottie's News

Months had gone past now, and Mum wasn't happy about me living at Dottie and Chris's. That bothered me if I thought about it too long, but not enough to do anything about it. *No way.* Nothing, not a top-of-the-range dirt bike, not a thousand brand-new pounds, *nothing on God's earth* would get me to live back at home again – *are you joking?*

I'd go and see Mum for a cup of tea, but out of duty more than anything, if I'm honest. I still wanted to see my brother and sisters, but now it felt a bit awkward, even with them. It was like we'd forgotten how to be with each other.

'So, is there any special lass in your life, son?' Mum was trying her best but, honestly, I wouldn't have been chatting about that stuff with her even if I had still been living there.

'Not really, no,' I said, conscious that now all my siblings were looking at me, interested all of a sudden.

There *was* actually a lass I was seeing by then, a friend of a friend of Murray's from town, and I'd fallen hard, but it hurt me even to think of her, because I could tell my Tourette's was going to bring it to an end any minute.

I waited for the piss-taking to start – this was where Sharon and Caroline and William would have laid into me, told me what a loser I was – but no one said anything.

They didn't even have a go at me any more, and even though I used to hate it when they did, I'd have preferred that – anything – compared to the formal, stilted way we were together these days.

I remember the throat-clearing and long silences, only broken by another tic from me – 'Twats!' – as we all sat there wondering what we could think of to say next. I'd be checking the clock on the mantelpiece – *how long before I can get out of here?* – and after maybe twenty minutes, I'd make my excuses and leave.

Mum would save it all until it was just the two of us, hissing to keep her voice low as she was seeing me out of the front door. 'It's not right, son – you know that, don't you? Living with another family?'

'I'm happy there, Mum. They don't mind having me, honestly. They like it; I help them out.'

'Don't be so naive, son. How can they like it? All that shouting and smashing stuff! They're using you. Can't you see? A dying woman in a wheelchair! They've got themselves an unpaid carer, haven't they?'

There was no point arguing with her. It was hard for her pride to take – I got that – so I just kept my counsel. She was always going to hate me living there, and if I went on about how much I liked it, she was only going to hate it even more. I could see it made her feel better to think of them as the baddies, and me as just stupidly naive. I didn't want to rub her nose in it; Mum was always on the edge of being able to cope with all that life had thrown at her as it was, and I felt like that would just push her over.

'OK, then, nice to see you, Mum. I'll pop in next week,' I'd say, and I'd leg it, as fast as I could, back to Dottie's.

I'd got into the habit of cleaning Chris's car. He'd never asked me to, but I was keen to do anything to earn my keep, and I needed to keep on keeping busy. After I'd been living there for a couple of months, I remember coming back into the house one afternoon, holding a couple of plastic bags bursting with all the rubbish I'd collected from it.

'Honestly, Chris, there'd be no room for anyone to sit in your car if I didn't sort it for you,' I said, waving the bags at him as I went into the kitchen, where he was standing with Dottie and Murray.

I could tell something was up as soon as I saw them. They never stood like that: lined up in a row, all proper, like some kind of awkward welcoming committee.

'What?' I scanned each of their faces in turn. 'What is it?'

'We've got something to tell you,' Chris said.

I went all dizzy when he said that – I'd always thought this would have to happen, any day now. 'Oh,' I said, thinking I might just fall flat on the floor.

I knew this had all been too good to be true.

'Where do you want this rubbish putting, then?' was all I could think to say.

They'd got together and had a chat, *of course they had* – and decided it was time for me to go.

'By the way, I found £2.65 in coins down the sides of the seats,' I said, pulling the money out of my pocket, piling it up, hands shaking, on the table, thinking, *What can I say next? If I keep on talking, maybe they won't say it.*

'You should take a look at your car, Chris. It looks brand-new inside – you wouldn't recognize it.'

'Davidson! Stop stressing will you, and look at me.' Dottie was smiling.

Smiling. That felt a bit heartless. She could maybe wait till she'd seen the back of me before looking quite so chuffed.

'I've no got cancer,' she said.

I went dead quiet for a few seconds. Everyone did as they watched me, waiting for the epic news to find its way in, past the messy tangle of thoughts piling in on me.

'What do you mean?' I said. 'I don't understand.'

'It's nuts, isn't it?' Murray said.

'But how can you have cancer, and then not have it?'

'They made a mistake.' Chris had his arm round Dottie's shoulders and was looking at her, grinning, as he talked to me. 'She has something called a hemangioma, don't you, love? It's a mass of cells on her liver, not, as they thought, a malignant tumour. Which means she's not going to die. Well, not just yet, anyway.'

'So that's it – we can stop being nice to you now, Dottie?' Murray was laughing, but I could see he'd been crying; the rims of his eyes were all pink like a guinea pig's.

I just stood there, waiting for a feeling to hit. I didn't trust good news. *Where's the catch?*

'Are they sure?' I said. 'How do we know, though – for definite – they haven't got it wrong?'

'The consultant called; he's absolutely certain. He was very apologetic,' Chris said, 'as he should be.'

'Dottie,' I said, 'I don't know what to say.'

'Well, that's a first, John Davidson,' she said, with a whoop of delight. 'You always have something to say!'

And now all three of us were hugging her, arms overlapping as we formed a scrum around her. I started crying, and that set off Chris and Murray again, and there she was stuck in the middle of us, whether she liked it or not.

'Do I need to be getting an anorak?' She was laughing. 'Or are you going to be pulling yourselves together any time soon? It's just my blouse is feeling a tad soggy now.'

'I got us a drink to mark the occasion,' Chris said, taking a bottle of fizz from the fridge. 'And Murray, get some music on, come on!'

Celebrate the wins – that's what Dottie and her family taught me. They don't come along that often, so make a thing of each and every one of them, stretch them out any which way you can.

26

Driving With Dottie

None of us were prepared for Dottie's reaction. We were all on such a high in the days that followed her misdiagnosis, so it took a while for it to sink in that she wasn't actually feeling it, like we were. She must have been trying her best to pull it out of the bag, because it was subtle at first, but after a while I could tell something was off with her, and it was an effort for her to keep jolly. It was like all of her bounce had gone.

I had wondered, where do you go, optimism-wise, when you're like Dottie – peak positive already – and then life takes a massive, great big unexpected turn for the better? What does even more upbeat look like? Was it even possible?

Turns out, maybe not.

I'd only ever known Dottie as a glass-half-full kind of person, and I'd come to expect her – rely on her – to look on the bright side of everything, sniff out that silver lining, scrape out the barrel if need be. This was how she'd been when she'd thought she only had months to live! I'd thought that was Dottie and she was set that way for ever and ever, so it threw me: this flatter, 2D version of her, who had to keep going to lie down all the time.

'It's to be expected,' Chris said, when I asked him what was up with her. We were in the kitchen, and he was arranging custard creams on a plate on a tray, next to Dottie's favourite mug. 'She put all that energy into keeping alive when she thought she was dying; I think she's lost her sense of purpose for now. It's important, isn't it? To have a sense of purpose. It keeps you going.'

'Oh, aye,' I said, playing that sentence over in my mind, wondering if that accounted for the lost feeling I had, too, as I poured in the milk.

I'd never thought of purpose until he'd said that, and the importance of maybe having some.

The end of college was fast approaching, and I had no idea what I'd be doing after that. *What was my purpose? Where could I find it? Could Dottie and me maybe find ours together?*

'It's been hard for her not working,' Chris said, handing me the tray. 'She's always loved her work.'

'Aye,' I said, thinking, *Don't jerk, Davidson. That's going to burn like hell if you do.*

'And then there's the money thing, isn't there?' I asked as he opened the kitchen door for me.

'Yes, there's that, too,' he said. 'That won't be helping, I don't doubt.'

The bank manager came knocking on the door the next day.

Dottie had stopped working when she thought she was dying. She didn't have a choice. Even though it had never been cancer, the condition she did in fact have was debilitating, and she'd needed a wheelchair. So, even if she'd wanted to, she wasn't physically capable.

She had life insurance, though, and as soon as she thought she didn't have long left, she'd booked a taxi and gone straight to see her bank manager, who became a good friend of hers – like most people who spend any time with Dottie. Everyone ends up loving her, whether they like it or not.

'Look,' she told him, 'I'm gannae die.'

Poor bugger, she told me, *he didn't know what to do with himself. He didn't know where to look.*

'It's all right, dinnae worry,' she said. 'I've got this life insurance – I'm worth more dead than I am alive. Will you let me borrow some money from it?'

He gave her five grand.

Dottie's mum was furious with her when she told her. Dottie's mum was furious about most things, though. That's the kind of person she was – one who waits to find something to kick off about, to prove her theory that all humans are idiots, and that life is against us all.

'Most people give things away when they're dying, Dottie,' she'd said. 'They don't buy things. That's not what people do!'

But Dottie took no notice; she'd only ever expected her mother's disapproval, because she disapproved of everything and everyone. She'd always been a harsh woman, Dottie said, *hard to the core.* Her verdict on me, Dottie told me years later, was that I just needed a short, sharp slap across the face to sort me out.

It amazes me that Dottie came from a mother like that. How did she know to be kind? Who taught her?

She spent the borrowed money on having nice times with her family, like her fortieth birthday, when she took us all out to a really fancy restaurant in a hotel. I'd never been anywhere like it before.

It was like the ones you see in films, with thick white table-cloths and all the different glasses, with piano music playing, and too many waiters, all dressed like they were going to a ball.

The kind of place I'd have hated ordinarily, except by now I was so much a part of this family – this warm, funny, loud unit of people – that it felt like we were in our own world when we all sat down at that table. I remember us just laughing, and I even managed to enjoy the food, with minimal spitting.

At the end of the meal, Dottie started larking about, making out she'd forgotten her purse. We all knew she was joking, but I don't think the waiter did.

'What do we do now?' she said. 'Are we going to have to do the washing-up?'

I think it was the way the waiter looked so awkward, and how he stumbled over his words, that set me off.

'We're all skint!' I yelled. *'We're as skint as a Jew's cock!'*

The man on the table next to us had just taken a sip of red wine, which he spat out, spraying it, coughing and spluttering, all over the spotless white tablecloth.

I'm not a racist – you have to believe me when I say that – but my Tourette's dredged up this terrible phrase, all the same, because that's what it does: it finds anything to provoke the ultimate shock and offence.

Adept at deflection, as ever, Dottie waved her purse in the air. 'I was just joshing with you,' she said to the waiter, handing him her card. 'And can you add on another glass of wine for our neighbour here?'

Dottie's borrowed five thousand pounds had all been spent by the time she got the all-clear.

'I don't know how to say this . . .' The bank manager was shifting from foot to foot at the front door, Dottie said later.

'Just say it,' she said. 'You want your money back, don't you?'

She was allowed to pay it back slowly – ten pounds a

month, or around about. It was going to take a long time, and she needed to start getting back into work. She was still unwell, so she began part-time at first, doing youth work again, and that helped with her mood as well as the finances, but she still wasn't completely back to being Dottie.

All of us in the family were on Operation Cheer Up Dottie. The consensus was that she needed to keep busy – nothing too physically taxing, but she needed to keep her mind occupied at least.

I don't know whose crazy idea it was, but I just said yes when she offered to teach me how to drive. *That'll keep her busy*, I kept thinking, *keep her on her toes. She'll be too scared and stressed out to worry about a sense of purpose with me at the wheel, I bet.*

What were either of us – what were any of us – thinking?

It went just as you might think that it would. The nervous excitement alone was enough to set me off. We were still in the close, and Dottie was driving as she explained what she was doing, and all I could think was, *Don't do it, don't do it, don't do it*, as I stared at the steering wheel. And then I did it. I lunged forward and yanked the wheel hard to the left. The car knocked down the bins outside Mr Cartwright's house, and there were a couple of curtains raised, and quizzical looks, as the neighbours saw Dottie laughing at the wheel.

'Don't worry, no harm done, love. Shall we leave it there for today?' she said. 'Nip out and pick up the bins, will you? Then we'll head back for a cup of tea.'

I had another appointment in Edinburgh with the therapist, and after the bus fiasco, Dottie said it might be best if she drove me up there this time.

'I can keep teaching you how to drive,' she said, 'just not with you at the wheel,' adding 'not yet', which I think we both knew really meant 'not ever', but it was too painful to think I might never be able to drive for either of us to actually admit it.

It was all going so well for a while. I remember us blethering away to each other on the journey and having such a laugh together, just like we used to. She was back to smiling with her eyes and doing her proper full-on belly laughs again. I was riding high, so happy to be cheering her up and relieved to see the old Dottie coming back.

'I'm slowing down now, Davidson,' Dottie said, giving me the running commentary whenever she did a driving manoeuvre. We were on a winding country road and coming to a corner. 'So look, I'm going down to second gear, now slipping down to first.'

'Yep, Dottie, I get you,' I said.

Then I heard the sound of a distant siren.

There's something about the sound of a siren that really gets to me. It's too much. I hate it when an emergency vehicle passes with its lights flashing and that blaring, unbearable noise. All I can think of is danger.

I waited to see if it was coming our way, and yes, it was getting louder and more urgent-sounding.

'Pull over, Dottie, will you?' I said. 'Quick!'

'All right, give me a moment,' she said, her eyes darting to the rear-view mirror. 'Let me find somewhere. Just keep calm, OK?'

'That bank of grass there – stop there. Hurry, Dottie, now!'

She veered off, just in time. A split second later and it would have been so much worse.

The tic came and I whacked Dottie hard in the neck.

She passed out, just like that, slumping forward at the wheel as the police car sped past us, oblivious.

My practical side kicked in before I could panic.

I turned off the engine, pulled on the handbrake, thinking, *Thank God college taught me basic first aid.*

I pulled Dottie out of the car. *What if I've killed her?* I was thinking. *What if she's dead?* I laid her on the damp grass and leant down to give her mouth-to-mouth.

Seconds later she was spluttering back to consciousness, shoving me off her as she asked me what had happened, where was she? I apologized to her again and again. *Dottie, you'll never believe what I just did to you.*

I wasn't even late for the appointment with the therapist.

Dottie had built in lots of contingency time. 'Not for mouth-to-mouth resuscitation, though!' she said, howling with laughter now, completely recovered. 'But you never know with you, John, do you?'

'I'm never going to forgive myself,' I said.

'Honestly, my darlin', don't worry,' she said. 'These things happen.' *Except they don't, on the whole, do they?*

'Let's just think of it as a good story,' she said. 'One of the many joys of living with you, John, is that you learn to expect the unexpected. Life's not boring with you around, and who wants to be bored?' she asked, screeching confidently backwards into a parking space. 'Definitely not me.'

As I was heading up the steps to the therapist's room, Dottie wound down the car window. 'Hey, John, do you know what? I think you knocked some sense back into me! I'm just sitting here feeling not too bad, if I'm honest. I think I'm more like myself. So thanks for that, love. I owe you one!'

I didn't care if she was just saying that to stop me feeling so bad; whether she really meant it or not didn't matter. Only Dottie could do that: find a way to turn being thumped in the neck while at the wheel of a car into a positive thing, just to help me feel less terrible than I did.

How do you not love someone like that?

27

Handyman

Dottie was made up. She'd just heard she'd got a new job, as a warden in a local old folks' home, an assisted living complex called Cornmill Court.

We'd all known she'd get the job as soon as her mate Tommy Trotter, the community education officer for Galashiels, had given her the nod that it was coming up. Not because he'd wangle it for her – he'd never have done that – but just because Dottie was Dottie and, *come on, who wouldn't give her a job?*

She'd been smiling non-stop, all day, since she'd heard. Dottie has one of those faces made for smiling. Do you know what I mean? Some people just do, don't they? Her whole face just radiates joy, and it makes you want to be right next to her, so you can bask in the glow of it.

Good news always had to be marked and made a massive, great big thing of – that was the law, like I've said, in Dottie's house. Any excuse to celebrate. At six o'clock, on the dot, Dottie had the brandy and lemonade out, and she treated us all to a takeaway from the Chinese, with extra prawn crackers, mountains and mountains of them.

Big change was afoot. We were going to be moving house. *Moving house!* My thoughts just whirled around my head in a jumbled-up mess when she told me that.

Dottie's new job came with a three-bedroom apartment on the complex, with everything, all bills included – which made it an amazing opportunity, not to be missed, Dottie said.

I was so much a part of the family by then that it wasn't even discussed whether I'd be going with them or not. It was just a given that of course I was.

I don't do too well with change on the whole, but this time, maybe because Dottie and Chris were so happy and relaxed about it, I somehow didn't get myself too wound up about it. I cheersed along with everyone when Chris gave a toast to Dottie and even felt a bit excited at the thought of it. It was impossible not to get pulled into the mood, with everyone high on the news, gabbling and laughing away as we fought over the last of the prawn crackers.

We all settled in happily to Cornmill Court. The apartment was part of a modern red-brick building on the grounds of an old church, and since Dawn had just moved out to live with her boyfriend, it was exactly the right size for us. Being surrounded by gardens was a real bonus, too – all that greenery and the birdsong soothed me and helped to calm some of the chatter in my head.

Dottie loved her new job, and she fitted right in from the outset. She's got such a natural way with people, being so easy and open and upbeat, that everyone – all her colleagues and the old folks – clicked with her straight away.

But the lost feeling I had was still with me. College had finished and I was missing everything about it, the friends I'd made, having structure to my day. I was missing the learning, too, now that I'd felt the satisfaction that comes from sticking with something and getting better, bit by bit, until I got it, and was even good at it. For so long, the only way for me to cope had been by trying to stop something in me, closing down a part of me – with limited to no success. The tics had kept on coming, but still it hadn't prevented me from trying. Reducing myself had been my modus operandi for years, until it had become second nature to me. I'd found it revelatory to *start something* in me, allow my brain to work in a different way, to open up and let new information in.

Now what? I knew it was time for me to get a job. It had to be done. I kept bracing myself to go down to the job centre, but the thought of what an interview would set off in me made me prickle with sweat, and I'd find any excuse to delay. The crushing exhaustion the haloperidol brought on didn't help with my motivation, either. Anything that took effort was easier to avoid. Even the thought of any effort made me want to retreat to my bed again.

It was too easy for me to sleep the days away, and when I was awake I was only sludgily conscious and so lacking in energy that just imagining leaving the house, let alone pulling myself together enough to impress in an interview, was all it took to make me bury my head deep under my covers.

'No thanks, I'm fine!' I'd yell at whoever was knocking on my bedroom door this time, asking me if I wanted a cup of tea, *and if I did, would I like to get myself up and come and sit with everyone?*

You need to occupy yourself with something. Dottie and Chris had a way of saying this to me which somehow stopped me from going off in a defensive strop. Anyway, I knew they had a valid point. I really did need to do something. In fact, I was desperate to, I just couldn't summon up the energy.

*

Dottie asked me if I'd ever thought about coming off the haloperidol.

She didn't think it was helping me at all, she said – it might be worth a go, that's all, just to see if I was better without it.

I hated all the side effects I had to endure with it – the sleepiness, the blunted feeling it gave me, all the weight gain – and I couldn't stand the way the dryness in my mouth made my lips stick to my teeth, making it difficult for me to talk sometimes. But it made me nervous, all the same, just thinking how I might be without it.

'Is it worth it?' Dottie said. 'All of that? Just to maybe give you a slight reduction in your tics? What's the worst that can happen? If you tic too much, you can just go back on it again, nae bother.'

What's the worst that can happen? I repeated to my reflection in the bathroom mirror, but still, I couldn't bring myself to do it.

'Aye,' I said, 'I'll give it a go, why not?' when Dottie asked if I'd come with her when she did the rounds of the old people's complex, her daily check of the residents. That felt OK to me, achievable, seeing as it wasn't too far to go, and I'd met most of the residents already, sharing the same communal grounds with them. And anything to delay that visit to the job centre.

'Maybe you could mend the odd thing for them?' Dottie said. 'There's always someone needing something doing. Might be an idea if you bring some of your tools, just in case.'

I was nervous the first few times I went along with her. My palms were all hot and slippery and I had to keep wiping them down on my trousers. I was convinced that older people were more easily offended by swearing, and the thought of having an outburst in front of them bothered me no end, sending me off in a riot of jerks and shouts and barks.

'I do nae want to upset anyone, Dottie,' I kept saying. That's how I imagined it: that I might actually reduce an old lady to tears with the shock of it, or maybe even set off a heart attack in someone, *you just never know*. I didn't want the weight of that responsibility. The thought that I might have someone's life in my hands, and not being a trained medic but a seventeen-year-old boy with just a spanner and a hammer and an Allen key to hand – *and really, what good would they be?* – was, to me, a very daunting, tic-inducing prospect.

Dottie has always had a way of calming me, though. She has this amazing, covert skill of convincing and cajoling – *manipulating*, I guess you could call it – and she does it with such subtlety and tact that most of the time I'm not even aware she's doing it. I always think she would have had a great career in sales.

Some of the residents had dementia, so Dottie would always take care to remind them who I was, and why I was with her, and that I had Tourette's, explaining every time exactly what that meant, even if I'd met them already. The odd eyebrow would be raised, once in a while, if I dropped the C-bomb, or asked to see someone's bollocks, or suggested having sex – that kind of thing – but for the most part my theory about the easily offended elderly was turned on its head. They all got used to me really quickly, and soon they were actually happy to see me.

'Ah, you have John with you – now there's a lovely thing. I just wanted a strapping lad to help me move a table in here. Would you come on through?'

It was good to feel useful, and I enjoyed the novel feeling of being appreciated, too.

I painted walls, I bled radiators, I hung pictures, put up shelves, learning how to do things, and get better at them, as I went along. When I was done, I might sit down and have a good blether and a cup of tea with a resident. Just seeing that I could connect and get on with new people helped me no end with my confidence.

Mary McDougal, one of the most elderly residents, took a shine to me, finding any excuse to get me to help her with something or other. She'd ply me with Wagon Wheels and Club biscuits, and endless cups of weak tea with a dash of milk, no sugar, even though I'd tell her every time, 'Strong and milky, two sugars, please,' when she asked me how I took it. I didn't mind. I liked her company. We had a right good laugh together, me and Mary.

When a part-time job of handyman came up at Cornmill Court a few months later, I didn't even hesitate. I just went for it.

I remember the shock and the happiness just pouring into me when I heard that I'd got the job. *I can't believe this!* I was thinking as I held on to my juddering kneecaps, gripping them tight, trying to force them to go back to normal as the momentous news sank in. *Finally! I'm officially employed.*

I couldn't wait to tell Dottie. I couldn't wait to tell everyone, to see the looks on their faces. I called Mum: *Yes, I know, it's brilliant.* I called Dad: *Thanks, yeah, I'm dead pleased, I'd hoped I was going to get it, like you do, but you know, it was never a given.*

This time, it was my choice. I got to decide how we celebrated, with any takeaway I wanted in the whole of Gala.

I went for Indian, and we all had extra onion bhajis – two each. 'Have three if you want – go on, knock yourself out, you deserve it,' Dottie said, getting her lemonade and brandy out again.

'Do you think everyone can stop getting new jobs for a bit?' She was laughing. 'It's just I'd been hoping for this brandy to last me for a wee while yet, and I'm already down to my last dram.'

28

Loony Bin

I was grateful to have the job. It really helped, like I said, to have some of the weight and the pressure of all that worry about what to do next lifted from me. *Thank God for it.* But still, it didn't stop this baseline anxiety that I had, buzzing away inside me, all the time, like the low-level hum of a fridge. Maybe because, great though it was, the job didn't feel like a permanent solution. I just knew that I didn't want to do it for ever.

I kept fretting about the next bit. I couldn't live with Dottie and Chris indefinitely. That thought preyed on my mind all the time. Soon I'd have to face the real world on my own, and I was all too aware – keenly, terrifyingly aware – that without the cushioning effects of Dottie and her family, the real world was not very likely to be kind to me.

I wasn't being unduly negative, just realistic, having been presented with no evidence – so far, at least – to make me think otherwise.

That's why the OCD really kicked in, I'm sure of it. OCD can be linked to Tourette's, but it's also exacerbated by stress.

At first the intrusive thoughts came every now and again, but before long they ramped up and began to take over. Soon, they dominated everything.

The thoughts had a theme: nightmarish and catastrophic – always a guarantee – involving people or pets I loved getting killed. The more shocking and upsetting they were, the more likely I was to repeat them. I remember it started with obsessive thoughts about my sister being knocked down by a car. It wasn't just fleeting thoughts, either, but a detailed account, like a clip from a film being played over and over in my mind. I'd replay the point of impact, watch her being hurled through the air, hear her landing on the road with a sickening crunch, see her lying there all covered in blood, horribly twisted and contorted, and most definitely, without any doubt, dead.

Dottie had a gorgeous wee dog back then called Ginty. I really loved that dog, like I loved all dogs, and soon my intrusive thoughts brought in Ginty. I'd be walking her, and I'd let her off the lead – *There she goes*, I'd be thinking, *look at that* – watching her running off away from me, straight towards the main road, and then into the path of an oncoming car. All the while, I'd be powerless, just standing there watching as she got crushed under the wheels. *My fault, all my fault*, I'd be thinking, walking over, looking down at her flat, lifeless little body. *Poor wee Ginty.*

My compulsions got worse around then, too. I had to keep checking the light switches, countless times, turning them on and off and on again, waiting for the noise of the switch to sound right to me, which meant a certain kind of satisfying click, with just the right weight and depth to it. The volume on the TV remote had to be above level twenty, which was loud – too loud for everyone else – but any lower and I'd start panicking that something really bad was going to happen.

I felt the need to kiss every lamppost that I passed now, and if I missed one, then I'd have to run back to do it. That, along with having to step on every single crack in the pavement, meant that going out of the house and heading into town became more stressful and drawn out than ever. It was like all of me was out of control now, and I couldn't rein any part in.

My compulsions began to make me hurt myself. If I was riding my bike, I'd think I needed to stick my foot in the spokes, and I'd do it, sending me flying head-first over the handlebars.

I couldn't trust myself any more. I panicked as darker thoughts made their way in, convinced that if I went near a bridge, then of course, without question, I'd have to throw myself off it.

I was tired enough as it was, and now I could barely sleep. I couldn't think straight. Dottie would find me sitting on the stairs, with my head in my hands. *I can't deal with this, I don't know how to handle what's going on in my head.*

She was always so kind and understanding, with her hugs and her reassurances. 'Not to worry, it's OK,' she'd say, stroking my back. 'We're going to get through this.'

'I don't think so, Dottie.' I couldn't stop crying. 'This is too much for me to cope with.'

'We need to get you some help,' she said. 'Now, don't be fretting – I know what you think of it – but I'm going to be calling Dingleton Hospital, just to get you a little support, OK? That's all.'

I thought of Mum forcing me to make the call to Dingleton all those years ago, and the dizzying, end-of-days panic that it had brought out in me.

Back then they'd told me to go and have a little sleep and book in to see my GP.

I'd escaped by the skin of my teeth, by a whisper – *for now, for the time being, maybe.*

I had an image of Enzo and the lads and me mucking about back in primary school, chanting, 'Loony bin, loony bin, who's going to the loony bin?' It was meant to be a stupid joke, that's all. *What would they all think now, if they knew it was me actually going to the loony bin? No joke?*

Because now the woman on the other end of the phone agreed with Dottie that, yes, I needed to come in and see someone, straight away.

I remember sitting in the back of Dottie's car as she drove me there, thinking how my twelve-year-old self would be losing his mind right now, trying to jump out of the car, banging on the windows to be let out, desperately bargaining: *Please, no! I'll do anything, just don't take me to Dingleton, I beg of you!*

Now, I just didn't care. *Just do it.* I was so desperate for help, *anything*. Whatever it took, wherever it was, whatever that meant, I couldn't have cared less. I just wanted to be freed from those horror-filled, head-frying thoughts of mine.

We'd cycled down the drive to the Dingleton so many times – me and my gang, when we were lads – and, out to chase thrills, waiting, always, till it was dark, to make it extra, full-on scary. So the sight of it was all too familiar to me.

As Dottie's car chugged down the driveway, past the wonky pine trees, casting zigzagging shadows across the lawns, I waited for the fear to kick in, some kind of reaction – shame, terror – as the massive, plain Victorian building appeared, with its covered porch and giant, wide chimneys looming down at us. They'd been made that big especially, I'd been told – by Enzo, so it must have been true – for burning the bodies after the nutters went on the rampage, like they did all the time, going crazy and killing everyone in sight.

I felt nothing. A part of me had shut down. *Maybe this is good*, I was thinking, *maybe this is the way to deal with everything from now on.*

They had an acute mental health ward in Dingleton, and I saw a psychiatrist in an office on that floor. I don't remember his name, but he was tall and angular with slicked-back hair and had that sharp, upright posture that comes from being really fit or really confident, or maybe both. I remember feeling intimidated, small and hunched up in comparison, like a frightened woodlouse.

'I'm going to be honest,' he said. Nothing positive comes after someone says 'I'm going to be honest' – I'd long since realized that.

'I don't know much about Tourette's syndrome, so I don't think I can be of any help to you.'

I felt that dull thud of recognition. *Here we go.*

Dottie wasn't having any of it. 'But we need help with the OCD. It's not manageable; John needs some support, some guidance as to how to deal with it,' she said.

'If I'm honest' – he was at it again – 'if he were to be admitted here, it just wouldn't work. John's presence on the ward would be too disturbing for the other patients.'

'Cocksucker!' I yelled, making him flinch and blink, then give a little grimace as if to say, *See what I mean?*

'So, what are you saying?' Dottie had her hands on her hips, and that set-jaw look that could reduce grown men – though sadly not this one – to gibbering wrecks.

'What I'm *saying*,' he said, shuffling his paperwork, sitting up even straighter, to signal that the meeting was now over, 'is that you need to book an appointment with your GP.'

Dottie was raging, all pink-faced with indignation. *It wasn't good enough. She wasn't going to leave it there.*

A lovely Spanish guy, a nurse who was in the meeting with us, offered to show us out.

'He's right,' he said as we walked through the grounds to the car park. 'If I were you, I'd go back and see your GP.'

'Everyone always says that,' I said. 'It's what people say when they don't know what to do with me. *Fobbing us off.*' I was too worn out to care about being polite.

'No!' he said. 'Listen! That's not what I'm doing. I think you need to ask about anti-anxiety medication, to tackle the OCD. Maybe you don't need to be on the haloperidol any more, either,' he said. 'I think it might be doing more harm than good.'

'That's what Dottie keeps saying.' I looked at her for confirmation. 'She knows about medication and stuff, don't you, Dottie?'

'Aye, I've been saying that for months now,' she said. 'But it's good to have the back-up from a medic. Dinnae worry, John, I'll book an appointment. We'll sort it.'

Mum wasn't happy as it was that I lived at Dottie's, so when I told her that the doctor had taken me off haloperidol, and now I was on anti-anxiety meds instead, she hit the roof.

'Whose idea was this? Was it Dottie's? She's not a doctor, son. You mustn't listen to a word that she says!'

'No, it was actually a medic who suggested it,' I said, but it still made no difference. When she blows, she blows.

'What are you thinking?' If her voice went like that – all

shrill – it was game over when it came to getting through to her. 'It calms you down! You'll be all over the shop without it.'

'I'm a zombie, Mum. If that's what it takes to be calm, I don't want it.'

It took guts for me to stand up to my mum. She just has that thing, that matriarchal power, that makes all of us, probably even now, want to please her.

'I've been years like this' – I tried to keep my voice steady and even – 'and guess what? I'm done.'

After two weeks of no haloperidol and a small dose of anti-anxiety medication, everything felt completely different in my head.

My mind was slower, but in a good, relaxed way, and the wading-through-treacle feeling had gone. My intrusive thoughts hadn't completely disappeared, but they were containable now, and I found I could brush them off more easily, instead of letting them cripple me.

I began to feel more like my old self. The 'can't be bothered' feeling had left me. I started offering to go into town, asking if anyone wanted anything getting from the shops. Murray took the piss out of me for being a keener. I was popping down to Iceland to get the tea, nipping to the off licence to get Dottie's mum her bottle of Cinzano. Murray could rib me all he liked; I didn't care. My confidence was coming back.

There were other positive side effects, too. The weight I'd been steadily putting on began to drop off me, my mouth stopped feeling dry, it was easier for me to talk and think without having to drag each sentence bit by bit from the fog that seemed to permeate my brain.

To top it all, despite bracing myself for it, unbelievably,

there was little to no difference in the volume and frequency of my tics.

'Can you believe it, Dottie?' I couldn't get my head around it.

'It doesn't surprise me one bit, John,' she said. 'It's a nasty drug, and you were on it way too long. I just think it's scandalous that no one took you off it sooner.'

'But the doctors kept saying I should up the dose,' I said, 'when I'd say I didn't think it was working.' A montage of all the meetings I'd had played in my mind as I slowly, bit by bit, recalibrated.

It was one thing to accept that doctors didn't always know how to help and had given me a drug that seemed to make no difference to me.

Now I had to wrap my head around *this*: that I'd been given a drug – *recommended*, *encouraged* to take a drug – that had actually made things worse, reducing *me*, not my tics, to a blunted, half-conscious version of myself.

29

Moving Out

I don't know if it was because Mum still resented me living at Dottie's – she was never going to change her mind about that; her resentment was *for ever and ever, amen* – and she was just desperate to get me out of there, or if she knew, like I did, that now I was eighteen and employed, the time had come at last for me to live independently. Most likely, it was a bit of both.

I was round at Mum's – it felt like Mum's now, my old house, not mine – when she told me she'd seen a wee bedsit was up for rent, in a block of flats not far away. I could apply for housing benefit, she said. She'd come with me, if I'd like, to look at it.

I remember feeling sick when she said it, and almost welcoming the sick feeling in. It was as if the wave of nausea had been waiting in the wings for this moment, because I'd known that this grim time was coming for so long and there was nothing, not one thing I could do to avoid it.

What could I say? It was the last thing I wanted to do, but I was too proud to show it, and I wanted to do the right thing, *the normal thing*. I knew I needed to become independent. Anything, even if it meant a shite, scary thing like this, to make me feel that Tourette's wasn't going to stop me living a life just like everyone else. This was what people my age did. All the kids I'd grown up with were doing it too, *moving out*.

I'd been prepping myself for this for ages now, trying to gear myself up: *Come on now, John, it'll be cool to have your own wee place.* Talking to myself like a coach in my head seemed to work for me. *It'll be grand, won't it? Not waking anyone up with the tics, getting Murray and the lads over for a beer . . .*

'Nice big windows, aren't they?' Mum said as we waited for the estate agent to show us round the bedsit.

'Aye,' I said, looking up at the eighties low-rise block of flats, thinking it looked a bit dismal, and that the windows looked normal-sized to me, and they could do with a good clean.

'Oh, that's a lovely bit of grass, isn't it?' she said. 'Nice to have a bit of green when you come out the door.' I nodded, watching her taking in the washing lines, the plastic toys left about, the fag butts littered around the bin.

'Yes, I've got a good feeling about this,' she said, with a tight little smile.

I knew it was a bedsit, so I wasn't expecting it to be massive, but I just couldn't believe how tiny the place was – or 'bijou', as the estate agent called it. Just one wee, sorry-looking room, with a partition for the toilet and shower room, and a bedroom with a galley kitchen at the back. *I mean, what am I meant to say about this?* I was thinking, trying my best to be positive.

'Aye, you're not wrong,' I agreed with Mum. 'It *will* look more homely with some nice wee pictures up, and a few things, you know, to make it feel like my own.'

'It's certainly got lots of potential,' she said, unconvincingly.

'OK, then. I'll give it a go,' I said. 'Why not?'

I tried hard to play down leaving Dottie's, pretending it was nae bother, and they all played it down, too. I was going to be going back for tea most days, as it was – so it would be almost like I hadn't gone, Dottie said, trying her best to convince me, as well as herself, I think, because I noticed her eyes were all watery and her cheeks had gone blotchy when she gave me a tight, trembly hug goodbye.

I really hated living in that bedsit. I never told Mum about the drug dealing going on in the social housing opposite, or the people kicking off in the street after closing time, and at night it was so badly lit around the flats that I didn't feel safe.

I tried to get on board with it, I really did, but there was no way around it: I just couldn't stand it there. I kept geeing myself up, telling myself how good it was to have my own place and some peace and some quiet at last, but it turns out there's nothing peaceful about quiet if you're anxious all the time and full to the brim with worry. All the quiet did was leave me with the racing dark thoughts in my head, with nothing, and no one, to distract me.

I missed my dog, Cassie, a gorgeous black Lab whom I'd got just a few months back. She'd been living with me while I was at Dottie and Chris's, but for now she was staying at Mum's. I'd have too much on my plate with Cassie as well, she said, so she said she'd have her till I'd settled in.

I'd been wanting a dog for ages, and I'd gone for an older one – on Dottie's advice – so she'd come ready trained. She was lovely, the easiest dog to look after. I kept calling

Mum, saying I was ready to have her, but I think Mum was loving having her too, because she was in no hurry to bring her back.

So it was just me, for the first time ever, with no Cassie, and no Dottie and Chris, no Murray, Dawn or Roddy or anyone.

I'd got so used to the background hum of their chatter and laughter, and their non-stop piss-taking, all the happy chaos of living with them, that I hadn't realized, until now, how much it soothed me. I didn't know what to do with all the quiet.

I'd go back to Dottie's every day for my tea, which helped for a bit, but each time I had to tear myself away from the warmth and the fun and the noise of their house, I just hated going back to my quiet, empty place all the more. I didn't feel safe. Not really. Not without them.

It wasn't long before some of the lads in the flats got wind that I was there on my own, and they started dropping round to my place all the time. Just a couple to begin with, but soon the bell was ringing every evening, and I was opening my door to find a group of them all crowded on my doorstep, waving their cans of beer.

'All right, John, fancy a bevvy?'

I was chuffed to have the company at first. 'Grand,' I'd say as they pushed past me. 'Come on in.'

It took a few days before the novelty was over and I was hating myself for being so naive. *Who was I kidding?* They didn't give a damn about me. I just had a flat, that's all, with no parents in it.

Soon my neighbours were having a go at me about all the noise, and the smell of the weed, and I was trying to turn the lads away. *Sorry, pals, not today, I'm just heading out* – but they'd push their way in all the same.

I wasn't joining in any more, but no one cared, so I just tidied up around them as they cracked open the beers and smoked their spliffs and cranked the music up louder and louder.

My brother, William, asked if he could use the flat once, to bring his mates over before they went out to a club. I was so dead keen to do right by him – anything to make up for all those years I'd kept him from sleeping – that I said yes without even thinking. 'I'll make myself scarce,' I said, 'go to Dottie's.'

I came back to find my place littered with fag butts, beer cans and pizza boxes, and the woman downstairs ranting at me about the music.

I really cared what people thought of me, so I was fretting all the time now about how much I was winding up my neighbours. Fretting is guaranteed to make the tics multiply, so they'd ramped up and adapted to their new environment, developed new ways to provoke.

Your neighbours hate you; they think you're a noisy bastard, I'd think, which would make me bang hard on the wall repeatedly, just to ensure that there was definitely no doubt about it.

I'd pass the couple from upstairs in the entrance and worry they'd given me a funny look, and so, back in the flat, I'd get the broom out and batter the handle against the ceiling.

The people from downstairs were giving me the evils yesterday, I'd tell myself, and then I'd stamp on the floor.

'Shut up, John, will you? Stop it, please!' they'd yell back at me, but that would just make me do it again, and again, hating myself, *cursing myself*, because this was the last thing – *honestly, if only they knew!* – the very last thing I wanted to be doing.

I had Cassie back with me now, so I had to be out walking her round the flats every day, and this stressed me out no end now that my tics were so bad. *Hurry up, just go now, Cassie, come on.* I'd be willing her to go, to get everything out as soon as possible, so I could hurry back to the safety of my bedsit and lock the door.

Every dog walk became a high-risk pursuit for me, because the harder or scarier someone looked, the more likely I was to insult them.

'Bunch of fuckers!' I shouted as I passed a gang of heavyset, wired-looking lads. 'Pair of slags!' I yelled at a couple of girls with massive back-combed hair, full of 'don't mess with me' attitude as they strutted past in their leather miniskirts. 'Fat cunt!' I ticced at the pierced-up, bearded Hells Angel revving his motorbike outside the off licence.

It was early evening, still light just about, and I was bringing Cassie back after a quick loop of the flats, when I saw two big lads I recognized from the social housing opposite, leaning against the wall near the entrance, dragging on the end of their fags.

'All right?' I said, because they were looking right at me.

'Took your time, didn't you?' the bigger of the two said, chucking his fag on the pavement. 'We've been waiting for you.' He ground the butt with the heel of his boot.

Now I could see the baseball bat propped up on the wall behind him. He picked it up and swung it, in daylight, and in public, with the casual ease of a known drug dealer, fully aware of his reputation as someone – with all good and proven reason – to be shit scared of.

I'd known this would be coming. *You can't go round shouting out insults in a place like this without someone, at some point, wanting to smash your face in.*

They had a weapon, and there were two of them, both built like bouncers, so it wouldn't have been my plan to provoke them. But then, he shouldn't have said it.

'Is that your ugly-arse dog?' The bigger lad was pointing the end of his bat at Cassie. 'I'll start with her, shall I? Give her a right good battering. Maybe that might shut your stupid face up.'

The rage I felt, like a blinding, bright white light, propelled me on to him.

'Fuckers!!' I yelled. 'No one *ever* insults my dog, do you get that?'

I remember pounding him with my fists, and the force of the bat whacking into my head, my chest and my back, over and over, and then out.

I was lying on the ground, that's the next bit I remember, with my lip all bust and swollen, blood stinging my eyes, and Cassie standing over me, licking the side of my face.

In the end it was Murray who called time on the flat. He was coming round to see me all the time – *spying on me*, he told me later, sent there by Dottie, so he could report back on how it was going. *Not well*, was the consensus. *Not well at all*.

'Dottie says you're to come back to ours,' Murray said. 'Just for a bit, till the council find you somewhere better.'

I was too knackered to think straight when he said it, and

so confused by my reaction – the push and the pull of relief and shame all mingling together – that I couldn't tell if this was good news or bad news, or what.

I wanted to move back, of course I did – *how could that not be better than this?* But the sting of disappointment I felt – *I'm failing at being independent* – just wouldn't permit me to be all right with it.

'OK, then,' I said, hating myself because I hadn't – I couldn't – make it work. 'Just for a bit, though, that's all.'

30

Langlee

I meant what I said. I really was hell-bent on not staying too long at Dottie's. It was too nice for me, that was the thing – way too cosy, like slipping into a warm bath, and I never was any good at getting out of baths, always topping up the water, staying in until my fingers went all pink and creased up with wrinkles.

I knew what I was like. If I wasn't careful, if I wasn't tough on myself, then I'd be wanting to live at Dottie's for ever – *why wouldn't I?* With every week that passed, it would only get harder for me to tear myself away. I could tell that the resolve I felt now, this burning feeling I had to lead an independent life, no matter what – just a normal, acceptable life; *is that too big an ask?* – could be buried all too easily in the comfort of life with Dottie, and then that'd be that: I'd never be able to find that drive to leave again.

I felt like I was in a holding pen – *waiting, waiting* – not daring to relax and enjoy myself too much, because any minute now it would be over. I was dreaming about it all the time, waking myself up with my tics, yelling out 'Fuckers! Bastards!' after another nightmare: Dottie and Chris booting me out in the dead of night, locking the front door on me. I'd be outside on the doorstep, shivering in just my pants, banging on the window: 'Please, Dottie, Chris, come on, let me back in!'

Dottie understood. She picked up on how I felt about everything. I've never needed to explain with her; she just knows. She could see the struggle I had with needing to do the right thing, and the turmoil that it set off inside me, because that right thing was still the last thing that I actually wanted to do. She knew just how to reassure and calm me, always finding a way to bring me back down whenever I got myself into a dither about it all. Endlessly patient, she sat down with me to fill in all the forms for the council, helping me to apply for another flat.

It didn't take long. Only months later, a new place came up for me, and now I was moving out again, a bit further away this time, to a flat on an estate in Langlee.

'Langlee's *miles away*,' I said, ticcing with the stress of it. 'Fuck Langlee!'

'Now, dinnae worry, John.' Dottie must have said that sentence to me at least three times a day. 'Langlee's going to be a great place for you. Remember there's that youth club Tommy runs? In the community centre there?'

Her mate Tommy Trotter was always busy with some kind of community project or another. He was a community education officer, so it was part of his job, but Dottie always said he took on way more than he needed to – *because that's just Tommy*, she said, *a decent, caring fella through and through*.

'I'll give him a call,' she said. 'I can ask if you can volunteer there if you'd like? He's been saying he could do with some help for ages now.'

'Oh, aye, yeah, maybe, I'll see,' I said, obsessing about the distance to Langlee. *Is it too far to walk back to Dottie's for tea? Will I be forced to take the bus? Please God, not the bus . . .*

'It might just keep you out of trouble.' Dottie was smiling. 'Keep you busy. You did say you want to keep busy, didn't you?'

She was right. Part-time work wasn't enough to occupy me, and it felt a wee bit mean to think it – it's not that I wasn't grateful – but I was a teenager still, and sometimes it got to me that I was working in an old folks' complex. It made me feel like I was missing out on things.

'It'll be good for you to be around some young folk, too. I think you need that, don't you?' Dottie said.

What did I say? She knows everything that's going on inside my head.

Langlee had a bit of a reputation – folk said it was rough – but it didn't take long to see it wasn't all that bad.

It was a big step up from my last place, though to be fair, that wasn't too hard.

My new flat was on the fourth floor of a pebble-dashed block – modern-ish – with wee balconies that looked out on to a green. There were cherry trees, too, bursting with blossom in the spring, and a wee park not far off.

It sat right by the main road that led up to the community centre, so nice and close to the place where Tommy's youth clubs were run.

I loved it straight away. After the bedsit it felt huge, and I was just made up to have a separate bedroom and a proper bathroom – that was class.

This is it, I thought. *This is independent living. Look at me go.*

I remember those first few days, heading out to work with

my head held high, nodding hello to folk, making eye contact with my brand-new neighbours.

They were all friendly and smiley, with no reason to hate me – not yet, not *ever* if I played it right. It felt good. *I* felt good. *New start. I love this new start.*

It didn't last. The buzz wore off way too quickly. *What goes up must come down.* I kept singing that song in my head over and over. It was being played all the time back then on some advert.

So what if my flat was bigger and better? It made no difference – that was the harsh reality. I was still ticcing away again, just like last time, banging on the walls, stamping on the floor, whacking like mad at the ceilings. I think I'd been kidding myself that the new flat meant a new me, convincing myself that the extra space would maybe calm me, bring on some Zen-like peace in my head. *No more tics.*

It's going to be different this time. I was always telling myself that. I should've had it printed on a T-shirt, a reminder of the endless, naive optimism I had, because I still had some faith – for some crazy, inexplicable reason – that life would get better, or *I* would get better, or folk would get better, *who knows?* It all amounted to the same fantastical thing.

I'm the neighbour from hell. The guilt and the shame of it ate away at me, because I knew by now these new neighbours would be hating me too, just like the last ones.

Before long I was scuttling off to work, head down to avoid the glares, hurrying past people, thinking, *Don't tic, not now, don't tic*, and shouting out even more with the stress of it.

'*I'm a paedo! Fuck you! Fuck the lot of you!*'

I remember the panic hitting me as the thought crossed

my mind: *What now?* There was no going back. Not this time. I couldn't run back to Dottie's again.

This is it now, I thought, passing a lamppost, stopping to kiss it, feeling sick with the certainty of it, *this is fucking it.*

I've got to find a way to stick this out.

'Go on, then,' I said to Dottie when I was back there for tea one day. 'Tell Tommy I'll give him a hand at that youth club if he wants me.'

I'd been chewing it over non-stop since she'd brought it up, mostly thinking of all the reasons not to, but I kept coming back to the same thing: I liked Tommy. I'd met him a few times when he'd popped in to see Dottie, and I'd taken to him straight away. He had that same natural, easy way about him. Maybe that's why the two of them got on. And any pal of Dottie's came with a Kitemark seal of approval, so I knew I could trust him.

Normally, the thought of trying something new would scare the shite out of me, but if I was going to try something, it may as well be with Tommy. Besides, the loneliness was worse. That kind of low-level, everyday isolation that gets right under your skin. It just made the fear feel daft by comparison.

Desperation's funny like that – it'll shove you out the door before you've even laced up your boots.

Dottie must have had a word with Tommy. Maybe she'd told him I can get a bit het up with new scenarios, especially when it comes to meeting new people, because I could see him waiting for me at the entrance of the community centre as I walked through the car park, his small, stout figure unmistakeable as he hovered by the door, waving to get my attention.

'John! Good to see you!' he said, smoothing down his ginger moustache, which looked redder than ever, spotlit by the bright neon outside light. *Where did that red come from?* I was always fascinated by his moustache. It didn't make sense when the little that was left of his hair was just a dark, mousey blond.

'Fuck off, you fat ginger cunt!' *I just knew that was coming.* 'Sorry, mate, no, I mean, hi Tommy.'

Tommy just smiled. 'It's grand you're going to help us here. Thanks, pal,' he said with a slap on my back. 'Next week you can come a bit earlier to help Stan, the caretaker, set up, but I thought it might be good for you to just come along for the first one, see what it's all about, eh?'

'Aye, nae problem,' I said, surprised by how relaxed I felt as I followed him into the reception.

'Nice new trainers,' I said. I'd clocked that he loved to be in the latest sportswear.

'Aye, I thought I'd treat myself – why not, eh?' he said, giving a little twirl to show them off, beckoning me to follow him to the hall. 'It's the senior youth club this evening, so we've got about forty-five or so kids from twelve to eighteen years old, all causing chaos in here.' He pushed open the double doors.

The swell of the noise, and the sight of all those kids, took me straight back to school, the *misery* of it.

That feeling. Back to that feeling. I was on the outside again, looking in from the sidelines, watching everyone, all these kids – the intimidating, unselfconscious ease of them – just being themselves, all together and the same, having fun.

Why did I say I'd do this? I was thinking. *What am I doing here?*

I started ticcing, just shrugs at first and yelps, and then I started shouting 'Fuck off!' repeatedly.

I was primed to apologize. That was how it usually went: I'd meet someone's stare, say sorry, then try to briefly explain. This time there was no one's eye to catch. No one was looking; they were all just carrying on.

'Just to let you know, John, I had a wee word with everyone before you turned up.' Tommy was leaning in to whisper. 'I gave the kids a bit of background about Tourette's, you know, explained what it was like, that kind of thing.' He was fixing me with this look he did, kind of half amused, like he was just about to break out into a smile. 'So it's OK, you can relax,' he said, putting a hand on my rigid shoulder. 'They'll nae be bothered, OK?'

I can still remember that moment, standing there with Tommy in that crowded hall, ticcing away, as I watched the kids mucking about, playing badminton on one side, football on the other, doing crafts on a table in the corner, and none of them, no one, reacting to me. I remember just how strange and how amazing it was for me to be able to tic like that, in public, in a place full of people, and yet not be the centre of unwanted attention, to feel no judgement for once – for the first time ever, it felt like.

Tommy was blethering away to me about what I'd be doing next week, the disco they'd be having, how I could set it up with Stan, and as I was nodding, taking it all in, I felt my body loosen, my muscles unclenching, bit by bit.

'Hey!' One of the lads setting up the football game was waving at me. 'Do you want to be goalie?'

'Aye,' I said, 'go on, then. I'll give it a go.'

'Sound!' he said, looking made up. 'Yeah, come join us then. Excellent!'

I remember heading back to my flat that night filled with this incredible, superhuman energy, buzzing and sparking like I'd been rigged up with electricity.

What just happened?

Walking wasn't enough for me. I couldn't contain it; I needed to use up all that power. *I've got to run to Dottie's,* I told myself, and now I was pounding along the pavement. *I could keep on running like this,* I was thinking, to the *scratch, scratch, scratch* of rough tarmac under my feet. *I could go a hundred miles an hour, no problem, just keep on running like this for ever.*

The kids had been nice to me. All evening. And when I say 'nice', I don't mean fake nice, I don't mean 'doing their best for Tommy' kind of nice, I mean proper, not-making-an-exception-for-me nice. I'd just spent three hours with all these lads and lasses who'd made me feel, in the best possible way, completely unexceptional. (Except in football, where I'd been massively exceptional, even for me; I'd saved three goals, making my team go nuts, piling on to me, shouting out my name, all punching the air, yelling, 'Yesss!')

I'd kept on waiting for the sly looks. I'd been ready and waiting for someone to shove me, or spit in my face, start calling me names – *something, any kind of kickback.* It hadn't happened.

What had just happened, I realized, was . . . absolutely nothing.

I knew it was down to Tommy. He said he'd explained Tourette's to the kids, but he must have done it so carefully and well, in a way that made sense to them. He got it. He understood what Tourette's was. He knew Dottie, he knew me, and that gave him an insider's insight, and he'd used it for good; he'd used it to help these kids get it, too.

As I got to the main road, I broke into a grin, and I just kept on smiling.

Here it is, I thought, seeing the opportunity outlined so clearly to me now.

I can start here, I told myself, my breath streaming out in front of me as I pumped my arms harder, desperate to see Dottie's face when I told her.

There are possibilities now. That's what it felt like, and I was full, brimming over, with the promise of them.

31

Youth Club

I was counting the days, and later the hours, and then minutes, until I could go back to the youth club again. Tommy had asked me to go back to help out on Sunday evening, which was four days away. *Not long*, I kept thinking, hoping I could kid myself to relax about it, *not long*.

It didn't work. Four days still felt like bloody ages away to me. That's just the way my brain works: anything that's not happening today may as well be in another lifetime.

Fuelled by nervous excitement, my mind had gone into overdrive, so the youth club was all I could think about, all I could talk about. Those four days took so long to pass. *Waiting, waiting, waiting. Come on!* I'm not sure who it was worse for: me, or Chris and Dottie. I knew they were happy for me, relieved I was finally fired up about something, but I must have driven them mad, jabbering on and on, and repeatedly, obsessively counting down how long I had to go, like a little kid in the back of the car on a long journey. *Are we nearly there yet? How about now?*

'I'm going to hand my notice in at work, Dottie.' I was up at hers for tea, pushing a forkful of her vegetarian bake around my plate.

'Slow down, Davidson, will you?' she said, pointing her

fork at me. 'You've nae even done the volunteering yet. Don't go getting ahead of yourself, OK? Do you nae like that, by the way?' She was nodding at my plate.

'Aye, it's no bad, Dottie, thank you,' I said, wishing I'd pressed harder to go to the chippy. I loved that Dottie was into cooking healthy food; I just didn't want to eat it, that was all. I'd take crispy cod on a nice pile of chips over this, any day.

'Trust me,' I said. 'I just know it's what I want to do.'

'It may well be, but just wait is all I'm saying. Wait and see how it goes on Sunday.'

Dottie knew what I was like, the way my optimism could set me up for a fall.

'Now come on,' she said. 'Get a wee bit more of that down you, will you? I reckon I've given myself RSI with all those vegetables I've been chopping. You'd better make it worth my while, OK?'

When Sunday evening finally came around, I got to the community centre half an hour early. Fretting all the way there – *what if I'm too early, what if no one's in?* This was the risk I'd always take, and the worry that came with it, which still was better, I'd learnt, than the stress that came with the fear of being late and what that would then do to my tics.

The lights were on in the community centre – *you're OK, John, you'll nae be standing outside like a lemon*, I told myself as I saw a man in blue overalls sweeping the parquet flooring in the foyer.

I wanted to knock, but my tic beat me to it and I shouted out 'I'm a paedo!' to announce my presence instead, which got his attention.

'Hello,' the man said, letting me in. 'You must be John. Good to see you.'

I nodded, biting down on the inside of my cheeks, trying to hold off any more tics until at least – *please God* – we'd got past the introductions.

'I'm Stan, the caretaker,' he said, putting out his hand to shake mine, but there was no way I could take it when all my effort was going into clenching my hands tight behind my back, clutching my fingers together, trying to counteract the tension building in my arm.

I managed a hello and a smile as I stood there, all rigid and awkward, fighting the massive, overwhelming desire that I had to hit him.

Stan was a small, slight man in his sixties. *If I hit him . . .* I didn't dare think, I didn't dare imagine. Any more thoughts about it would surely only make it more likely to happen.

'Tommy said you'd be coming,' he said, like he hadn't even noticed I'd skipped the handshake. 'Come on, I'll show you what's what.'

'Skinny cunt!' I yelled as my arm broke free and I swung myself away from him, smashing my fist into the wall.

Stan didn't react. Instead, he calmly explained what he'd like me to do, showing me the table in the foyer where I'd sit to sign the kids in and take their money when they arrived.

'Fucking dump of a place!' I yelled. 'Sorry, Stan, I didn't mean that. *Stinks like shite in here!* No, not that either, sorry.'

Stan gamely carried on, held up a hand and shook his head as I apologized again, to let me know: *No need.*

'Badminton's for pansies!' I shouted as he went through the equipment cupboard with me, where all the nets and the balls and the shuttlecocks were stored, all the stuff I'd be setting up.

Back in the foyer again, Stan took me to the coffee bar area, where I'd serve the kids snacks and drinks.

'Aye, I'm fine with that,' I said. 'I've worked in a van before, served coffee and tea and stuff . . . *Spunk for milk!*'

'Would you come and help me set up some chairs?' Stan said by way of reply.

'Yes,' I said, relieved to be finally put to good use. 'Yes, *I'd love to.*'

I'm thinking now of what it was that made that first evening work so well for me. *Work like magic,* if I'm honest, because it was so much better, in every way, than I'd even dared to imagine it might be.

The kids had respect for me. This was a massive, unexpected result, something that had never even crossed my mind. Why would it? I'd never been respected before. But somehow there I was, a youth worker now, in a position of authority, and I could see that really meant something to the kids as they filed in one by one – 'Hiya, John' – all polite and friendly, with their pleases and their thank-yous.

Yes, a few flinched when I let out a shout, or twitched, but none of them laughed at me, not one. I think there was something about me sitting behind a table, too, and taking their money, which made them see me as an adult – a grown man – which I hadn't ever recognized, or even felt, that I was.

They were almost shy of me, that first evening. *Shy of me!* But as time passed, they got bolder and more curious.

'Why do you swear when you tic, John? Do you mind me asking?'

'We were just wondering why you're so loud when you tic?'

'Did you always do it? Or did you wake up one day and that was it?'

The questions kept coming, and I was happy to answer them as best I could – *this is just what I wanted* – as I sorted out the speakers for the music, handed out balls, put up nets. I was grateful to be busy while I was doing it, which helped me to keep calm, so the tics died down loads, making it so much easier for me to explain to them.

Tommy dropped in to see how it was going.

'You doing all right, then, Davidson?' he shouted over the music, ducking as a ball flew over our heads. 'Not too mad for you?' He smiled.

'Aye, it's amazing, Tommy. This is . . . *everything*,' I shouted back. 'And I love it being mad.'

'You do nae find it too much, I can tell,' he said, patting my shoulder approvingly.

'I was really nervous, Tommy,' I said, 'in case it was like school, you know, but it's not formal, I'm not disrupting anyone here, I'm not getting on anyone's nerves.'

'Aye,' he said. 'Besides, I dinnae think anyone could even hear you ticcing above all this racket if they tried,' he yelled. 'You might want to go and turn that music down a notch or two. I'd like to come out of here with my eardrums intact, if that's not too much to ask of you.'

I laughed. 'Aye, Tommy, your wish is my command, sir,' I said, heading to the CD player.

'Constant Craving' was playing – k.d. lang, her lovely, heartfelt voice somehow cutting through all the noise of the kids and filling the room, even through the crappy, tinny wee speakers.

I'd loved that song from the first time I heard it. I just got it. I knew what that constant craving felt like. I'd lived with it for years and years now, that all-consuming driving force, that desire that takes over everything, because all I wanted, all I yearned for, above all else, was acceptance. I just wanted folk to accept me.

That OCD thing I had, about flicking the light switch again and again until it made just the right kind of click? Well, that's how I'd describe that first evening.

It just clicked – and not just any click, but *the right kind of click*. I relaxed, properly, at last, because that craving that had been dragging at me for years was just gone.

There was no need for it.

Look at this, I thought as I stood in the hall, with kids all around me – and now I wasn't on the sidelines; I was right there, in the centre, in among it all.

It's happening, I thought as a lass pulled on my sleeve.

'Excuse me, John, would you help us find some coloured paper, please?'

'Aye, it's Jenny, isn't it? Nae problem, follow me. I'll go and get it for you.'

I'm a part of something, I thought. *Finally.*

32

Community Centre

Dottie's always been my sounding board on all matters under the sun – that's just how it's always been with us. I was twenty now, and living my own life, but still, I'd be ringing her all the time, asking what she thought about this and then that, the new jacket I might buy, the recipe I could try, the latest lass I thought I might have a soft spot for. I'd run everything and anything past Dottie. *Do you like it? How should I do this? What about that? What do you reckon?*

'Dottie, have you got a sec? Can I ask you . . .'

'Aye, Davidson, go on,' she'd say, with a long, over-the-top sigh, but I think she loved being thought of as the oracle of all things. At least, I *hope* she did . . . I should maybe check with her . . .

That morning, though, the morning after I'd done my first volunteering at the youth club, I didn't even think to ring Dottie to double-check what she thought.

Anyway, she'd already given me her two pennies' worth. I should wait before handing in my notice – that's what she'd said. *And you've not long had Tilly; don't have too much change in one go.*

My gorgeous dog, Cassie, had sadly passed a few months back, and I had Tilly now, another black Lab, who I'd had from a puppy this time. She was working out brilliantly, but I was still getting used to a new dog, and a bit anxious about getting things right with her.

So if I'd called Dottie to ask whether *right now* counted as waiting, she'd only have said, *Do you nae think you should hang on a wee bit longer?* I could be impulsive – she knew that – so she'd try to get me to err on the side of caution. It didn't matter. Right now, as far as I was feeling, caution could go shove its finger up its jacksy.

I didn't need Dottie's opinion, because for once, for the first time since God knew when, I realized that I knew what I thought. I needed to leave my job immediately. Something just felt right. I needed to be helping out at the community centre. *From now on. For ever. This is it.*

Feeling so certain about something was such a weird and novel thing for me. I was so used to my mind being constantly muddied by this mass of conflicting thoughts all day long – honestly, it knackers you out when you have a head like that – and this *knowing feeling* felt so clean and clear and precise to me, such a welcome break from all that.

It takes me a while to get started in the morning, but that day I was up and out of bed the minute I woke up, all itchy to get going, shoving on my tracksuit bottoms, and my favourite, softest-feeling sweatshirt, pushing my feet into my trainers by the door. No time for coffee or breakfast, *no way*. I was in that much of a hurry to get down to Cornmill Court and be done with it, so I could begin the next bit. *This massive next bit of my life.*

'Come on, Tilly, we've got to go,' I said, forgetting her lead, then the poo bags, locking the door, opening it again, back and forth – *keys, where's my keys now?* – all light-headed and distracted by this churned-up, momentous feeling. '*Fuck!*' I ticced, head jerking, as I finally left my house. '*Fuck, fuck, fuck!*'

Self-doubt used to take up a lot of my headspace back then. On a good day, it was like I had a bully in my head; on a bad day, it was more like the devil. Maybe it was part of my Tourette's, or maybe it was because of it. Who knows? It's not something I even noticed at the time, so I never thought to question it. They were just my thoughts, and my thoughts were the facts of the matter.

'I'm a jobless wanker!' I ticced as I left Cornmill Court, having just quit my job as a handyman. 'I've done it. I can't believe I've actually done it, Tilly, can you?'

Tilly waited patiently by my side as I stopped to give a lamppost a kiss.

'Come on girl, good girl,' I said, shouting '*My dog's got worms up its arse!*' as the pretty lass from the pound shop walked past.

The sky was a flat sheet of grey as I walked back to Langlee, and it was half-heartedly raining – that mist of constant drizzle, so light you can barely see it, the kind of rain that gets you wet slowly, by stealth, so before you know it you're soaked right through.

Would it be OK to turn up to the community centre all wet, with my hair all flat on my head? I wondered. *I'll look like a right spanner by the time I get there*, I thought, *like one of those Lego men with clip-on hair.*

I've just left my job. I should be feeling bad by now, I told myself, waiting for the doubts to flood in. *What the fuck have you done, Davidson?* That kind of thing. *You're a right stupid idiot. You'll nae get another paid job again* – the usual mental beating-up I'd subject myself to.

But nothing came. There was just this empty space in the place that they should have been. I remember the feeling of the fresh, wet air as I breathed in, wondering about that, thinking, *maybe this is what they call peace of mind.*

Tommy had said I could help at the community centre that day, *in the daytime.* There was a playgroup to set up for, he said, then some kind of networking event later on, so anything, even an hour or so, would be a help to Stan, and yes, he'd said, nae problem if I wanted to bring Tilly.

'Come on then, girl, let's go see Tommy, shall we?' I said as we waited to cross the road. Tilly looked up at me, adoringly, with that open-mouthed showing-all-her-teeth expression she did that made it look just like she was smiling.

It was her cute face that did it, and the surge of love that followed, which made the tic swing into action to kibosh it.

'Go on, Tilly!' I shouted, pointing towards an oncoming car. 'Go on!' And, obedient as ever, she went for it, sending me lunging after her, yanking her back, shouting 'No!' as the car raced by, its driver angrily sounding the horn.

'So sorry, my darling.' I buried my cheek in her head. 'I don't mean to. I'll try not to do that again. I love you. You know I love you, don't you?'

She just looked up at me, with her smiley face, loving me back as much as she ever did, none the wiser.

Life can get too comfy at times. Do you know what I mean? With Tourette's, every day can be fraught with risk, so it had made sense for me, I guess, to try to keep things as safe-feeling and easy as possible. For a while – for too long – I'd been keeping my head down, avoiding things that might stress me out, living a pretty quiet and comfy existence with my nice, low-key, part-time job at the old people's complex, and tea at Dottie's most nights. It was good – and necessary for me, too, in many ways – but it meant there was nothing to challenge me, either.

I knew that helping Stan out in the day was going to test me. I'd get het up if I thought too much about it, but I was hungry for it, too, dead keen to work as hard as I could. I wanted so badly to prove myself, not just to me, but to Tommy and Stan, *to the whole of Langlee.*

The community centre was the heart of Langlee, so everyone and anyone came through those doors at some point. *So many people.* I found it overwhelming when I started, all the hellos and how-you-doings. *I'm John, working here with Stan. Aye, nice to meet you.* All the while, I'd be trying to stop the tics from coming. *Bellend!* Doing all I could to contain myself. *Fucking knob-head!* Biting my lip, holding down an arm. *Jelly tits!* Breathing deep – *calm, keep calm, keep them down.*

Back home, at the end of the day, I'd call Dottie and she'd try to stop me from spiralling. 'Come on, Davidson, you've been banging on for ages now about wanting to meet people, haven't you?'

'Aye, I guess so,' I said, rubbing my temples, my head pounding from all the effort of it.

'You've been feeling out on a limb and wishing you were in the thick of it,' she said, 'and you can't get more in the thick of it than the community centre, can you? Be grateful – see this for the opportunity it is. You're a right lucky bastard!'

'Thanks, Dottie, aye, you're not wrong.'

'You've just got to relax and get into it. Would you like me to give you some reiki? Would that help?'

'Oh, no thanks, Dottie,' I said, way too hastily, ticcing, *'Christ, no, not that hippy shite!* I mean, thanks, that's a lovely offer, but you're all right.'

'You'll be fine once you get to know everyone,' she said. 'It's just when they're strangers you struggle.'

She was right, of course. She's always right.

Gradually, it got easier as I got to know people and, bit by bit, they got to know me.

I could tell from the start that I wasn't causing the usual shock and offence – thanks to Tommy having a word again, I don't doubt – because, just as it was with the youth group, almost everyone seemed to know exactly what to expect with me.

'Hiya, John, you're looking well today. Are you all right if we go in the hall now?'

'Aye, Janice, *fat heifer*! Sorry, yes, I got the chairs all set up for you, and I put some extra trestles in there for you too this time, *slag*! *You fucking slag!* Sorry, Janice, sorry about that.'

'Ach, it's nae bother,' she said, smiling. 'I can but dream! I'm sixty-five, so those days are, sadly, well and truly over now.' And we both started laughing. 'Oh, and thank you for thinking of the tables,' she said as she went into the hall. 'What would we do without you, eh?'

What would we do without you? I'd replay that sentence over and over in my head at night if I couldn't sleep, just to remind myself that I was doing all right, that I was actually doing OK.

Before long, you couldn't keep me away from the centre. I was up there more or less every day, helping Stan out with all the caretaking jobs, then back again in the evenings for the youth club. Tommy would have to have a word with me sometimes, tell me to rein it in. 'John, it's great that you work so hard, but, lad, you're nae getting paid, so go home, have yourself a bit of life once in a while now, OK?'

What a massive difference a bit of confidence makes.

Now I was feeling a wee bit better about myself, it seemed to me like everything, *everyone* appeared better to me, too. I didn't even notice it happening at first, but as my confidence grew, my behaviour began to change along with it. Instead of rushing out of my flat with my head down, I started looking my neighbours in the eye again, smiling and saying hello to them.

Guess what? My neighbours turned out to be lovely, and it took a while for me to believe it, but it turns out they didn't hate me at all.

I was happy to stop and blether to everyone, even Wendy and Shaun, the couple downstairs who I was sure I'd been driving mad with my ticcing.

'*I'm a noisy wanker! I'm your neighbour from hell!* Sorry, no, sorry, Wendy, I just wanted to say I dinnae mean to do that banging on your floor. I try not to, I promise, I'm so sorry.'

'Oh John, dinnae worry about it.' Wendy was laughing. 'The first time, I thought the roof was falling in,' she said. 'So I was like, *oh, thank God*, when Shaun said he reckoned it was just you having a wee bang with your broom. Don't you stress about it, John. If you need to have yourself a wee bang, you just go for it!'

The relief that I felt when she said that. The *gratitude*. I'm not into the hugging and kissing and stuff, but right then, I wanted to scoop her up and hug her and kiss her and say,

Thank you, thank you. You have no idea, you have no clue what your words have just done to me! It was like a tight string had been cut inside me, and I could feel myself straightening up again. Shame can be such a weighty feeling. You really notice that when you feel it lifting away from you.

There was a lovely lass, Karen, a single mum with two kids, who lived in the flats opposite me. I'd bump into her in the shop sometimes and, now that I was being a bit bolder, I was brave enough not to rush off, and I'd stay and have a natter with her about this and that. We got on straight away. She liked to have a laugh, like me, and she had that laid-back, happy-go-lucky way about her. I've always been drawn to people like that, people who aren't easily offended, because, let's face it, me and anyone who takes offence – no way that's ever going to happen.

Karen and I got close quite quickly. I'd go round to her flat for a cup of tea, and to watch TV, or we'd go for a wee trip downtown.

She worked at a local restaurant, and before long I'd be babysitting her kids when she had a shift.

'Are you sure, John? You dinnae have to do this, you know?' she'd say. 'I can always ask my mum.'

'I'm happy to, honestly, Karen,' I'd say, which was true. *'You're beautiful!'*

'Aye, John.' She'd just giggle when I said that. 'I know I'm beautiful,' she'd say, half joking, but kind of not, because that was true, too – she was.

I'd started to develop feelings for her. I think it would have been hard for me not to: she was gorgeous and funny and easy company; everything, really, that I wanted in someone. But all this made me increasingly anxious, which set me on edge and made things more difficult and tense for me.

I'd been through this before, when I was seventeen and I fell for a lass who I saw on and off for a while, but in the end my tics were too much for her. I couldn't deal with that heartbreak, I didn't want to feel that way ever again, so I'd steered clear of any relationships since then, hating what it did to my head, all the stress and the panic it brought out in me.

Imagine what it's like having Tourette's when you take a shine to someone. It's good to take it slow, isn't it? Wait to see if you get a sign that maybe they might like you back. It's a bit of a game at first – you don't want to be too keen, too fast, in case they're not into you, and even if they are, being too full on from the start could easily put them off.

With Tourette's there are no cards for you to keep to your chest. There's no holding back. You just lay them straight on the table.

'*You look like Linda Lusardi!*'

I was never offensive to Karen, but I think I'd have found it easier if I had been. If I'd ticced '*Slut!*' or '*Whore!*', I could have hidden my feelings for longer, and I'd have just said *Sorry, I didn't mean that*, and we'd have had a laugh about it, no harm done.

The problem was, I couldn't ever say, *Sorry, I didn't mean that*, after I started to have feelings for her. '*I love you! Karen, I love you!*' Because I did mean that. I did.

'I've been keeping my eye on you, Davidson.' Tommy liked to say dramatic things like that, to make out I was somehow in trouble, but I'd been at Langlee for six months by now and I'd got to know his ways, and I was wise to it.

'Oh aye,' I said, 'just the one eye?' Then ticcing, '*You bong-eyed twat!*', my words echoing round the car park.

I was up a ladder, at the front of the centre, and Tommy was holding it for me as I had a go at cleaning out the gutters.

'You're a hard worker, I appreciate that, and I can see you've got a talent for the youth work,' he said. 'You're a natural. I knew you would be, too.'

'Aye, I enjoy it, Tommy,' I said, passing him down a handful of wet leaves and twigs. 'I feel like, you know, I know what to say, *you fat ginger nonce*! Not that, sorry – you know, when I'm not ticcing, I know what to say to the kids. I can see when someone maybe needs a wee bit of attention. Like I did. I know how that feels.'

'Aye, I see you doing it,' he said. 'You're always looking out for the ones being left out. I hear the way you talk to them,' he went on, 'and you listen to them, too. You've got a real way with the kids. I'm impressed with you, pal.'

'Thanks, Tommy. That's nice of you to say,' I said, glad to be up the ladder and looking the other way so he couldn't see my cheeks burning red, and the massive stupid grin I couldn't wipe from my face.

I'd been starting to think that I might actually be OK at the youth work, but thinking I was OK at anything didn't come naturally to me, so it was only in a *maybe, we'll have to see* kind of way. But Tommy had just confirmed it and made it feel like a real, actual thing to me.

'I listen to the way you talk about your Tourette's,' he said, 'and how you explain it to the kids, and they're taking in your every word. I think Dottie's right.'

'About what?' All the praise had made me go a bit dizzy, so I got myself down the ladder now, just to be safe.

'I think you can do more,' Tommy said. 'I know you go to those Tourette's Support Group meetings?'

'Aye,' I said, 'every month. It's been great for my confidence. The folk running it have been asking me to maybe give a talk or something, for the new members coming in.'

'Well, why don't we think a bit bigger?'

'How do you mean?' I said, brushing the mess of mulched-up leaves I'd thrown down away from the entrance. *'You're so fucking boring, spit it out, man!'*

'Aye, you're spot on,' Tommy laughed. 'Dottie and I were thinking we could organize a weekend with the Tourette's Support Group, for the kids with Tourette's and their families.'

'OK?' I said, turning to look at him.

'We haven't got much further than that yet,' he said. 'That's why we need to talk about it. But how I see it is, you'd be the lead for the weekend, and it would be up to you how you'd want it to go, of course, but I was thinking you could give talks, use your experiences to give guidance to these families,' he explained. 'Tell those kids like you what you say to the lasses and lads at the youth club, you know, explain how you find living with Tourette's, how you cope with it.'

I was quiet for a moment, waiting for the chatter in my head to quieten down – the tics trying to break free, all the doubts battling with the pride and elation, the great big tangly mess of it. I couldn't speak when my head got like this.

'Shite idea! You're thick as shite, Tommy!' I yelled. 'No, sorry, I didn't mean that. I mean, that sounds amazing, Tommy, scary as hell, but yes, amazing.'

'We could run workshops, and help the families start to feel part of a community,' Tommy said, 'so they don't feel so alone with it. I just remember you saying that to me once, how you wished you didn't have to feel so alone with it. It's only an idea for now, just a seed I thought I'd plant in that head of yours. Have a think.'

'Aye, Tommy, can we have a chat about it some more, but inside with a cup of tea? I'm freezing out here,' I said, shouting *'Freezing my tits off!'* as I saw Rosemary from the council getting out of her car.

No, I told myself, *don't. Don't say it.*

Dottie had just let slip to me that she had a hunch that Rosemary might be Tommy's secret girlfriend.

'Tommy's got a micro penis!' I shouted after her. 'Sorry, Tommy, I dinnae mean to.'

He rolled his eyes at me, shrugged her an apology.

'And gonorrhoea!' I shouted. *'You do nae want to have sex with him!'*

33

Blue Lights

I left my flat, all full of it, ticcing away with excitement. '*Karen! Beautiful Karen!*' I shouted as I raced down the stairs. '*I'm going downtown with Karen!*' Then, '*Fuck me, Davidson, you numpty!*' which wasn't a tic, I'd just looked at my watch. It was ten a.m. and we weren't even meeting till eleven.

'For fuck's sake! Tilly, what are we going to do with ourselves now, eh?'

It was one of those dead peaceful mornings, all sunny and lovely and quiet, and Tilly was pulling on her lead, raring to get in among it all.

'Come on then, girl,' I said. 'Do you want to go get some squirrels?'

The park was empty, which was just how I like it, so I sat on a bench for a while, taking in the sunshine and listening to the blackbirds chirping away.

I only notice the birds when my mind quietens down. A rare thing, but when it happens, it's just lovely.

Maybe now's the time, I thought, *while I'm nice and calm. Maybe now I can have a wee practice of my speech.*

'Hello, everyone, thank you for making the journey to be here. My name's John . . .' I began, and then the words just flowed and I didn't falter, not for one second, because I knew exactly what I wanted to say.

By the time I'd got to the end, I could tell from the way Tilly was looking at me that she thought the same thing as me.

'I know, you're dead impressed too, aren't you, my darlin'?' I said as I patted her head.

The first weekender with the Tourette's Support Group was happening in Perth the next weekend. Twenty-five families had been asked if they'd like to take part, and all twenty-five had said yes. Tommy and Dottie and I had been planning it for weeks, and even though I'd get tied up with nerves when I thought about it too much, that certainty I had was still with me, and I just knew that I had to do it.

I was pumped up, and feeling really chuffed with myself, by the time I walked to Karen's flat. *Look at me go,* I was thinking, *I'm amazing*, whistling 'Eye Of The Tiger', boxing the air in time to those massive big drumbeats.

'Hey, John, who do you think you are?' Karen shouted down from her open window. 'Rocky Balboa?'

'Aye, Karen, you're spot on!' I yelled up to her, ticcing, *'Juliet! My Juliet, I'm your Romeo!* Are you coming, then? Are we going into town?'

'Give me a sec, let me find my purse. Aye, I'll be right down.'

We were playing that game as we walked into town, the one where you whistle a tune and the other one has to guess what it is.

'Could you no tell that that was "Careless Whisper", though?'

'And you're blaming me, are you, John? Do you no think that might just be your godawful whistling?'

And we were carrying on like that, laughing and mucking about, and I was flying, thinking, *This is the best morning*, grinning away, thinking, *I didn't think life could be like this*, and then we turned the corner into Kenilworth Avenue, and it went like that bit in a film when a record's playing, then the needle scratches and the music comes to a screeching halt.

'Oh God! Oh God!' we were shouting now, and running towards the man lying in the middle of the road, all battered and covered in blood, with his bike half on and half off the pavement.

I could tell who it was from the second I saw him. That small skinny body, those blue overalls – it could only be Stan.

'Stan, Stan, you're OK,' I said, shaking with shock at the sight of him. '*You're fucking awful, pal,*' I ticced. '*The state of you!*'

His face was streaked with blood, and the knees of his overalls were ripped and bloody, and he had bits of tarmac sticking all over him.

'Are you John?' he said as he tried to sit up.

'Aye, Stan,' I said, 'it's me.'

'I'll be fine,' he said as I tried to make him comfy. 'I'm fine,' he kept saying as Karen called an ambulance. 'Honestly, I'm fine. You don't need to do that,' he said, wincing with pain.

Stan wasn't fine. Maybe it's a generational thing, or maybe it was just Stan, who was never one to make a fuss about anything. It turned out he'd sustained serious internal injuries in the accident, and he was going to need weeks in hospital to recover.

A day or two later, Tommy called to say he'd like to have a word with me in his office. I remember wanting to be sick when he said that, because anyone saying they wanted a word with me in their office just took me straight back to school, and all I could think was, *I'm in trouble.*

'We're going to need someone to stand in for Stan while he's off,' Tommy said, 'so would you fancy taking on the job of caretaker, Davidson?'

'Do you mean it, though?' I said, knowing how Tommy liked to joke around with me.

'Of course.' He was laughing. 'You've been working your arse off for nothing for ages,' he said, 'so it's about time you got paid.'

'I'll be shite!'

'Now, I'm no going to lie,' Tommy said, 'there's a few on the board, they've got issues, you know, with you having Tourette's, so you're just going to have to prove them all wrong.'

'I can do that, Tommy,' I said. 'I'd be delighted, *I'm fucking made up, man!* Thank you, for having the trust in me, *you fucking eejit, you're gannae regret it!* No, you're not, I'm going to make you proud, I promise you.'

'We both know you can do it,' Tommy said. 'And between you and me . . .' he added, tapping the side of his nose.

Don't say 'between you and me', I was thinking. *Please never say that to me.*

'Between you and me,' he said again, never missing a chance to be dramatic, 'you're the best caretaker we've had.'

'Best caretaker!' I yelled as I rushed outside to call Dottie. *'I'm the fucking best caretaker ever!'*

Dottie went nuts when I told her. She was all *oh my God, oh my God, I can't believe it,* calling Chris, getting him on the phone so I could tell him all over again. It was like I'd just said I'd won the Nobel Prize.

'Hey, Karen! It's me, John. Can I come up?' Twenty minutes later I was talking into her intercom, ticcing *'I'm a rapist!'* as she buzzed me in, *'I'm a fucking rapist!'* as I raced up the stairs, desperate to get to her. *She'll be impressed with me now,* I was thinking as I got to her door. *Yes, she'll be dead impressed with me now.*

'I've got a job!' I yelled, the minute she opened the door. *'They've given me Stan's job!'* Wishing I could have waited, just until I was in her flat, strung it out for a second or two at least.

'John, no way! That's amazing! Come here,' she said, pulling me in for a hug.

'No, you're amazing!' I ticced, thinking how lovely she smelt, just like roses. *'I love you!'*

'Fraser, do you know John?' Karen said, turning back as she pulled away from me.

There was a man sitting on her couch, in the place where I usually sat.

'No, we've not met,' the man said, smiling as he stood up and held out his hand to me.

'Wanker!' I shouted as I forced myself to shake his hand. 'Sorry, I've got Tourette's,' I said, thinking, *I want to die, I may as well be dead,* thinking, *I hate you, I fucking hate you, you good-looking bastard.*

I ran back to the park, burning all the way, jerking and ticcing, *'Fuck! Fuck! Fuck!'*, hating myself, hating my stupid fucking Tourette's, mucking everything up again, like it always did, ruining my life.

The park was busy now, but I sat on the bench again,

because I was there, and what else could I do? And I just sat there with my head in my hands, and I cried and I cried and I cried.

'Are you OK there, John?' Wendy from downstairs was standing over me, frowning with concern.

'Aye, Wendy, no bother, I'm fine,' I said, thinking, *Fuck me, I'm just like Stan, saying I'm fine when I'm not. When I'm fucking broken inside.*

I shouldn't have gone out that night. It was stupid of me – I was in no fit state – but when I'm in no fit state, it's not always easy for me to make the right decisions.

Murray had heard about my job, and he'd sorted a night out for me with some of the lads we played football with. Me going to pubs was still a new thing. I'd only just got myself in the right place to be able to deal with being out in public at night, but I wasn't in the right place now.

I should have just gone round to Dottie's, or got myself to bed, had an early night and waited for all the anger and the massive, great heavy sadness to pass, instead of pretending it had never happened and obliterating the feelings – obliterating myself – in pint after pint of beer.

I was still a mass of tics when I got to the sports bar off the square, jerking and ticcing all over the place. That's how it goes when I'm upset – they become like a physical manifestation of my pain.

It was heaving in the bar, jam-packed, with folk spilling out on to the pavement, and pints sloshing all over the place as people tried to squeeze themselves to the bar. Even surrounded by my mates – and they were all out tonight, about eight of them – I was feeling edgy and paranoid.

'I can see what you're doing, John,' Murray said. 'Stop looking around, will you? There'll always be someone – just ignore it, shut it out, man. Come on, we're here to enjoy ourselves.'

'Aye, I'm trying,' I said. 'But those lads over there' – I raised my pint to a table by the door – 'can you nae see they're all laughing at me?'

'Turn your back to them. Don't waste your time on ignorant arseholes,' Murray said. 'Let's remind ourselves *you've got yourself a job, mate*! Come on! Cheers to that!'

Maybe if they hadn't started mimicking me, I'd have left it at that, but now I was watching all these men twitching and jerking, all pissing themselves laughing, and I was drunk, and it was too much. I couldn't stop myself.

Murray tried to pull me back, but I shook him off, and then I was standing there at their table.

'I can see you're taking the piss out of me.'

They all stopped and looked at me. 'No, we're not,' one of the lads said, but he was smirking, they all were, and that fucking enraged me.

'Dinnae deny it,' I said, as Murray pulled at my arm and said, 'Hey, hey, hey, John, leave it, will you? Just let it be.'

'You do nae know what it's like for me,' I said. 'I've got Tourette's; I cannae help it. It's hard enough for me already, without you lot taking the piss out of me.'

What was I expecting? *Oh, sorry, mate, we've behaved like arseholes, our mistake, please can you forgive us?* They just pissed themselves laughing.

The humiliation – that horrible, straight-back-to-school feeling – made me tic with my arm and it shot out, just missing the fella's face.

I didn't have a chance to explain. He was on me, and we

were scrapping in the doorway, with Murray and everyone all yelling and trying to pull us apart like we were a couple of fighting dogs.

'I don't think Tommy's best pleased with you,' Jenny on reception said.

It was a couple of days later, and I was arriving at work early, like always.

'Oh aye,' I said, ticcing, *Shite, I'm getting a bollocking now!*'

Jenny was always one for playing things down, so I knew that when she said he wasn't best pleased, what she meant was he was off-the-scale raging mad with me.

Tommy was like that: calm as anything for most of the time, but, my God, if he lost it, you were best off running for the hills.

'Can you tell me, Jenny, does he know?' I said, ticcing, *I'm gannae be locked up in the clanger! For the fight! I'm a fucking fighter, don't mess with me pal!* Is that why? Does he know about me being taken to court?'

But it was too late for her to answer, because there he was, striding towards me. *Face like a slapped arse!* I ticced.

'Can I have a word with you, Davidson, in my office?'

There it was again, that dread-making sentence. Except this time, I knew I was right to be bricking it.

Tommy didn't sit at his desk. He stayed standing, looking out of the window, as he spoke to me. 'So, John, we've got the weekender coming up on Saturday, haven't we?'

I hated the way his voice sounded, all cold and flat, with no heart in it.

'Aye,' I said, my head hanging with shame. *Hey! Hey! Paedo!*'

'If you want to continue working with the Tourette's community, and doing youth work, if you want to be working with people, you can't have assault charges hanging over you.'

He must have looked round and seen the tears streaming down my face, because his voice softened then. 'You do know that, John, don't you?' he said.

I nodded and bit my lip, scared to answer in case any more tics came out.

'There will always be ignorant people, John. You're going to have to learn to find a different way to deal with them. What's the point in getting angry, eh?'

'*Pot and kettle!*' I ticced.

'Where does that get you?' Tommy said. 'You do nae want to get a reputation.'

'*You're nae the boss of me!*' I ticced, but I took his point all the same. He was right.

34

Weekender

We were on our way to Perth for the Tourette's weekender. Tommy was meeting us there, so it was just me and Dottie in the car, blethering away, Dottie doing her best, I think, to distract me with chat as she drove us through the beautiful Fife countryside, with its rolling hills and massive big skies, and mist rising all over the shop. I love a rolling hill, so I was taking photos through the window, trying to capture them with the fancy new digital camera Dottie had given me for my birthday, saying, 'Ach, well,' every time I checked the screen. They were blurry as fuck.

'I'm gannae really enjoy this journey on the way back,' I said, 'when I'm not scared out my wee tiny mind.'

'Dinnae fret,' Dottie said. 'Just remember, everyone coming just wants to hear what you have to say; they're not there to pick you apart.' She patted my knee. 'You've just got to be yourself, put it out of your head, don't think of it.'

Don't think of it, don't think of it, I said in my head, picturing myself standing up in front of all those families – *twenty-five times how many? Three or four, that makes . . . oh my God, like, a hundred people* – imagining myself standing up in front of them all. 'Pissing my pants!' I shouted. 'I'm gannae be pissing my pants!'

The roads were busier now, and it was all wide lanes and fast-moving traffic whizzing past as the massive Forth Road Bridge rose into view ahead of us.

There was a lot to take in, and I was taking in every single bit: all the cars – lots of red cars today, for some reason – the river way down below us, the wee boats – a blue one, a white one – and the other bridges – *too many bridges, what the fuck? Why do you need that many?* – one to the left of us, one to the right of us, and here was our bridge now, coming up, right in the middle. *I dinnae want to be hemmed in*, I was thinking, feeling myself getting wound up, winding tighter and tighter.

'Shall we no take a break now, Dottie?'

'Aye, soon, not yet,' she said. 'Let's get us over the bridge first. I cannae stop here.'

My hyper-observational skills extend to people as well; I'm always looking for visual clues that help me to tell what they're feeling. It's like a sixth sense, Dottie's always said, which comes from having Tourette's, I think, and always being primed to look out for danger.

Right now, I could tell that Dottie was petrified, and she was nae going to tell me. But she didn't need to – it was her white knuckles that gave it away.

'Are you afeard, Dottie? Do you no like heights?' I said, feeling my heart start to knock in my chest. Dottie wasn't meant to be scared. It was OK for me, but not her. *Otherwise what? Otherwise there was no hope for any of us.*

'No, no, I'm fine, John, I'm fine,' Dottie said, shaking her head, still gripping the wheel. I couldn't take my eyes off her knuckles . . .

'You dinnae like heights – I can tell, Dottie. Just tell me, just say!'

'If I said I'm fine, John, I'm fine! Will you listen to me?' she shouted.

I don't like Dottie to shout at me. It's not what she does, and the stress of that set me off.

'*Don't!*' Dottie was screaming now. 'John! *John! What are you doing?*'

I'd opened the passenger door as she was driving. *Do the worst thing*, my tic was telling me, so I was leaning out of the car. *Do the worst, most dangerous thing that you can.*

Dottie was screaming, having to keep on driving, with cars in front of us and behind us, as I hung on to the top of the open door and twisted round to face her through the windscreen.

'Get in!' she shouted as I held up my camera, managing to snap her, eyes wide, mouth open, mid-scream, before she yanked me back in, with one hand on me and one hand on the wheel, keeping the car on the road somehow.

'Why, Davidson, *why?*' she said, all sweaty and flustered, with her hair all over the place.

'You're afeard, Dottie. Why did you nae tell me?'

'Yes! I bloody hate heights!' she said. 'But I'm nae stupid, am I? I wanted to keep that from you!'

She was mad with me, and I hated that, and I tried so hard to fight it, gripping my hands as tight as I could to my seat, but the upset had set off a compulsion inside me, challenging me to top what I'd just done. *Go on, you can do it, you can go one better*, the voice was telling me. So I did. I went one better.

I leant forward and put my hand over her eyes.

I hadn't realized Dottie's voice could go that high. I remember the sound of her scream ringing through the car as I held my hand there, looking at the white van in front of us, thinking, *Will we smash into the back of it? Or will we go over the edge? Which will it be?*

'Oh my God, thank God,' Dottie said, with a wail of relief, as I released her just as we left the bridge.

'I thought we were dead,' she said, trembling all over, struggling to hold the wheel as her hands were shaking so much.

'I cannae drive. I've got to pull over,' she said, screeching into a parking place by the side of the road, yanking on the brakes.

'Dottie, I dinnae know what to say,' I said, following her out of the car.

'Nothing, John, don't say anything.' She held up a hand. 'Leave me be for a minute, will you? I just need some time,' she said, leaning over the bonnet and putting her hand on her chest, taking in some deep breaths. 'OK, now pass us my fags, will you?'

'I dinnae know how we're going to get back,' she said once she'd finished her cigarette, 'because I'm telling you now, I'm nae going over that fucking bridge again!'

And then somehow – God knows how – we were laughing.

'Did you get a pic of me?' Dottie said. 'Go on, then, let's have a look.'

We laughed even harder when I showed her the photo. 'Oh my God,' she said. 'The look on my face! Wait, just you wait till we show Chris!'

When we set off again – with my right arm wrapped up tight in the seatbelt now – everything felt a lot lighter. Dottie kept saying she was just grateful to be alive, and I think that sent her into some weird kind of high that lasted for the rest of the journey.

Maybe it was Dottie back to being Dottie, maybe I'd just used up my last drop of adrenaline, but now all my tension had disappeared, and I didn't feel nervous any more. All that fear, any doubts, had just left me.

The weekender was being held in an outdoor centre deep in the Perthshire countryside, and the last leg of the journey there was just beautiful. Perthshire's known as big tree country, but it's not just the trees – all of it's massive, kind of extravagant, in a show-off, peak-Scottish-countryside way. It's all supersized forests and craggy cliffs and deep valleys, with this vast, flat, wide river snaking through it, so clear we could see all the clouds and the blue sky reflected in it.

'Hello, everyone, thank you for making the journey to be here. My name's John Davidson,' I said, thinking, *Finally, I'm actually saying it. I'm doing my fucking speech.*

'I have Tourette's, so I know what it's like for you,' I said, scanning the kids' faces, their wee hopeful smiles, finding myself blinking back tears.

'*Fuck!*' I ticced. '*Fuck you all!*'

'Fuck! Fuck you too! Go fuck yourself!' came a torrent of tics from the kids with coprolalia.

'Well, at least I know you're listening to me, eh?' I said to a ripple of supportive laughter.

'The Tourette's Support Group has been a vital source of support to me over the years,' I said, 'helping to inform me, and giving me strategies to deal with my Tourette's. Now it's my time.' I looked up from my notes. 'I want to pass that information on to you.' I paused as I waited for the applause to die down and the riot of tics that accompanied it, all the shouting and yelping and whistling.

'For so long, you will have felt like the minority, but I want to say that right here, right now, you are the majority . . .'

You know those massive big moments in life, when something feels so momentous in that 'I can't believe this is happening' kind of way that you almost can't enjoy it, it's just that over-whelmingly good, and you don't want it to end, because when it's over you think nothing will ever feel this good again? It's like you're mourning it being over before it's even finished. That's how that first weekender was to me.

Everything about it just worked. I never needed to worry about how it was going – even me, with my full-on observa-tional skills – because right from the start, it was so obvious it was running exactly as we wanted it to. Better, maybe, even than that.

It was such a strange, bittersweet feeling I had as I stood watching the kids, all strangers to each other just a day or two ago, chatting and laughing together, ticcing freely away, getting bolder and more confident as they scaled trees and climbed ropes and did zip-wires. 'Go on, don't be scared, you can do it!' – egging each other on all the way.

It made me so happy and proud, but a tiny bit sad for the wee lonely twelve-year-old me. I knew how much I would have loved this as a kid, how much I'd needed it. I could see how different things might have been for me, if only I'd had something like this.

I kept thinking of Mum and Dad as the weekend pro-gressed, and how much they could have benefited from this, as I listened to parents sharing their experiences in the group discussions, comparing notes. *Yes, I know what that's like; we had that same thing too.* I saw their tears of relief – *someone else gets it; it's not just me* – watched them all laughing together – *I had that happen, too. My God, I wanted the ground to open and swallow me right up!*

Parents were coming up to me and Dottie, and Tommy, shaking our hands. They'd not seen their kid this happy in so long, they said, telling us how good it was, what a relief it was, too, for them all to meet other families.

Was there going to be another weekend? Could they put their names on a list? They knew someone else – could they come along, too, to the next one?

'You're always going to come across ignorant people,' I said, in my closing speech. 'And trust me, I know what it's like. It made me self-conscious. I used to worry way too much about what people thought of me. I'd be watching out for them laughing at me, mimicking me, taking the piss,' I said, scanning the crowd to find Tommy, who was at the back, leaning against the wall with his arms crossed.

'But where does that get you, eh?' I said. 'As a wise man once said to me' – exchanging a wink with him – '*it's him! That ginger-bearded prick at the back!*'

'Guilty as charged!' Tommy shouted, grinning as he raised his hand.

'You need to find a way to deal with it,' I said, 'and dinnae fret about what other people think. Tourette's is a part of your life, and once you accept that, you can live it as best you can.'

'Hey, Davidson! What do you think you're up to?' Dottie shouted when she saw me getting into her car.

'What are you on about?' I said, buzzing and full of it all, as I pulled the seatbelt across me.

'I know you did brilliantly,' she said, opening the passenger-side door. 'I know they all loved you, but don't be getting too big for your boots, OK?'

'Eh?' I said. *'You're no fucking making any sense to me!'*

'Out you get,' she said. 'Back seat only, if you're to be getting a lift home with me. Call me uptight, but I'd like to get home alive, if you dinnae think that's too much for me to ask.'

35

The Big Talk

In early 2006, a woman called Sophie Dow got in touch with me to invite me to be part of a conference she was organizing – 'The Social Brain', which was to take place in Glasgow.

It sounded like a really big deal. Forty of the world's leading specialists in neurobiology, psychiatry and child development were coming to give talks on the theme of sociability, she said. There would be all kinds of aspects to it, including neuropsychiatric conditions. Would I be one of the keynote speakers and discuss Tourette's syndrome?

I said yes, straight away. I don't think I really knew what I was letting myself in for.

'Are you happy with your speech?' Dottie said.

We were in Dottie's hotel room, the night before my talk. Joining the other speakers downstairs for a meal wasn't an option, so we were sitting side by side on her bed, waiting for room service.

'Aye, it's not too bad,' I said. In fact, I was being deliberately modest – no one likes a show-off, after all – and actually, I was pretty sure that I'd nailed it.

The talks I'd been giving at the Tourette's weekenders had

been going down really well, and I was getting better each time, so by now my confidence in my public-speaking ability was sky-high.

'Go on, then.' Dottie was getting out her fags, settling in. 'I'd like to hear it.'

I remember feeling really chuffed with myself once I'd read it out to her – I thought I'd done a grand job – so I took her silence for stunned admiration.

'Well?' I said. 'What do you reckon?'

Dottie took a long drag on her cigarette before she answered.

'John, this is a really big event – you know that, don't you? There are going to be hundreds of people listening to you, from all over the world.'

'Aye,' I said, 'of course. No need to scare me, Dottie. I'm trying to keep myself calm here.'

'I think you're pretending again,' she said.

'What do you mean?' I said, feeling my saliva dry up, the air going all cold in my mouth.

'You always present as if you cope just fine, don't you?'

'Well, that's what people need to hear,' I said when I found my voice, which was lost for a few seconds in the shock of it.

'But you don't always cope, though, do you? There are days when you bloody struggle, when you need some help,' she said.

I couldn't answer. This was so far from the reaction I'd been expecting. My mind was taking time to compute. I thought she'd come along to cheerlead me all the way.

'What about those days that you lie on my couch?' She wasn't going to leave it there. 'When you can't lift your head? When you won't leave the house?'

I could feel the fury building inside me. I didn't need to be reminded of this, not hours before I was about to do the biggest speech of my life.

'Why are you saying this to me, Dottie?' My skin was prickling, which only happened when I was a seeing-red kind of mad.

'You're in a position now where you've got all these people – lots of young people, too – all looking up to you, and that's great,' she said.

Keep it coming, Dottie. Go on, then, break me down.

'But I think you have a responsibility to be honest with them, don't you? You have to be positive, too, I agree, but I think it's important to tell them the whole truth.'

Her words stung me so hard she might as well have hit me round the head with a crowbar. No, scrap that – been there – this was worse.

'*Fuck off!*'

I've shouted at Dottie to fuck off many times, but this was the first time it wasn't a tic.

'I'm looking out for you too, you know, John.' She didn't seem flustered one bit. 'I listen to you on the phone and you always say "nae problem" to anything that's asked of you. You're always so keen to present as "can do", and I love you for it, but sometimes you have to be honest and say, "I'm actually struggling a bit today."'

'FUCK OFF, I said – didn't you hear me? I'm nae doing it. I'm never doing that!' I shouted. I remember trying to slam the door behind me as I stomped out of her room, but it was a fire door with one of those door closers at the top, so that didn't work.

I lay on my bed and stared at the ceiling. *I can't believe I told Dottie to fuck off*, I was thinking, shaking all over, as the red light on the fire alarm blinked back at me like an angry, reproachful eye.

After a few minutes, when I'd calmed down a bit, I got up, and I rewrote my speech.

Dottie opened her hotel room door before I'd even knocked on it. 'I could hear you out there ticcing,' she said, leaning in to give me a hug.

'You were right,' I said. 'It wasn't honest. I've put it all in now. I'm going to say it like it is. Like you said.'

I hadn't been prepared for the scale of the event. This was probably for the best, as I doubt that I'd have slept for weeks if I'd known just how massive the auditorium was, and how many people would be there. Every seat was filled, and there were hundreds of people all sitting waiting for me to speak. I was grateful I only had seconds to take it all in before I went up on stage.

I tried not to let the panic overtake me. Thankfully, Dottie was sitting directly in front of me, so I spoke to her when I gave my speech. I barely ticced once I got going, and my nerves disappeared. I even stopped reading my notes – I just spoke what I felt. I can't really remember what I said.

I couldn't believe it. I got a standing ovation at the end of it. I had to fix my eyes on Dottie to keep myself steady. She was smiling and crying at the same time, shaking her head, holding her hands high as she clapped harder than anyone.

This is good, this is good, this is good, I kept telling myself. *Don't freak out.*

Dottie really didn't need to say it, because I could see it, I could *feel* it radiating off her, but she mouthed, 'I'm so proud of you,' at me all the same.

Just in case I'd not picked that up, and it hadn't been so glaringly, heart-warmingly, best-moment-of-my-life-so-far obvious.

36

New Pal

It was December 2009 and I was in my sitting room, down on all fours, hiding from view, because there was a man standing outside my house, wanting to see me.

I've never been one for surprises, so when I heard my doorbell go and peeked out of my window to see a stranger standing there, it set me right off.

I won't answer the door to someone I don't know. Even when my friends come and see me, they have to let me know exactly what time they're coming. If I have visitors, I like to be prepared and revved up, ready and waiting at the window.

A stranger turning up with no prior arrangement meant I didn't know what to do with myself – which meant I had to call Dottie, so she could tell me exactly what it was that I should do with myself.

'He's still there,' I was whispering into the phone, just in case he could hear, thinking, *Be quiet, John, be quiet, be quiet*.

'How can you tell,' Dottie said, 'when you're down there on your hands and knees, like a numpty?'

'I just had a wee check,' I said, patting Tilly, who was lying next to me, 'and he's standing in the close, just looking up at my house. Dottie, what does he want from me? *Arse wipe!*' I ticced. '*I'm hiding! In here! Come and get me! I'm hiding from you!*'

'What does he look like?' she said.

'Dark close-shaved hair, well built,' I said. 'Looks like he maybe does weights and stuff . . . *Arnold Schwarzenegger!*'

'Ah. Not Dave, then.'

'Who's Dave?'

'Elsie's son, the plumber? Remember? I told you, I gave her your number to give to him when you said your boiler was playing up.'

'I don't know,' I said, scratching my scalp with the stress of it. 'What does Dave look like?'

'Well, put it this way: like someone who's ne'er seen the inside of a gym,' she said, laughing.

I heard a car door shutting, an engine revving. 'I think we're OK. *I think he's gone, Dottie,*' I said, getting to my feet, cautiously poking my head above the windowsill.

'Do you think it was maybe that fella we're meant to be seeing this afternoon,' Dottie said, 'at the centre?'

'Paul?' I said. 'I dinnae think so. It's only just gone ten, and we're not seeing him till later. And anyway, how would he know where I live?'

Dottie and I were meeting someone called Paul at the community centre after lunch, a guy from Berwick who'd got in touch with me via Tourette Scotland after a documentary I'd just been in, called *Tourettes: I Swear I Can't Help It*, had aired on TV.

He was watching it at home with his wife, he said, when she muted the TV and turned and just looked at him, and they both had the same eureka moment. 'I think you've got Tourette's,' she said.

'I know,' he said, 'me too.'

He'd put his tics down to nerves at first, he told me when we chatted on the phone, or maybe grief, he said, because they'd started when he was at his pal's funeral. His pal had died by suicide and he was feeling all guilty about it, fretting he hadn't been there enough for him, and each time he thought that, he twitched. His tics had built up from there, he said, and now he was swearing and saying all kinds of things, and he wasn't sleeping at night.

'I really need to meet you, John,' he said, ticcing, '*Hey! Hey, hey, hey!* Will you take a look at me? See if you think I've got it?'

I was anxious about meeting Paul – just a wee bit wary, you know, not really knowing the first thing about him. I asked Dottie if she'd come, and she was up for it, and then Tommy got wind that I was meeting someone and said he'd make sure he was knocking about at the centre, keeping an eye out, just in case we had ourselves some kind of nutter on our hands. I didn't think he sounded too bad on the phone but, like Tommy said, you just never know.

Dottie and I could hear all the whistles and shouts before we saw Paul, standing waiting for us at the entrance of the community centre, shifting from foot to foot.

'You were right, Dottie,' I said. 'It's him, the same guy who was up at my house – *casing the joint*! *Fucking casing the joint!*' I ticced.

'Were you no at my door earlier on?' I said, stopping a good distance away from him.

'Yes, that was me!' he said, looking dead pleased with himself, instead of guilty or sorry like I wanted him to.

'I wasn't sure if it was the right door or not. *Fifty pence!*' he shouted, bending one arm above his head and putting his foot on his opposite knee, standing there like some big, muscly ballerina. 'Then, when no one answered, I went and hung around in town. Sorry, I'm not good at waiting. I was a bit overexcited and keen to see you, that's all.'

'How did you find where he lives?' Dottie said, opening the door for him, pointing him towards the cafe area, where Tommy was busying himself moving chairs about.

'I freeze-framed the documentary,' Paul said, 'and I zoomed in on John's house, saw the number, stuff like that, and I worked out where it was from there.'

'*Fucking stalker!*' I ticced, choosing us the table nearest the exit.

'Fucking wanker!' he ticced back.

'Fuck off!'

'Fuck you!'

'Fuck your mother!'

'For Christ's sakes!' Dottie said, rolling her eyes. 'Will you listen to the pair of you?'

'Well, Paul, I dinnae think there's any doubt in my mind,' I said. 'You definitely have Tourette's, and you can add in echolalia and coprolalia to the mix as well.'

'So that's tea for everyone,' Tommy said, bringing a tray to our table, 'and we've got KitKats and Twixes if anyone fancies, and I think we've got a couple of Fudge fingers left, too.'

'*Fucking fudge packer!*' I ticced.

'*Fucking finger licker!*' Paul ticced back, and we went into a volley of tics, back and forth, all *fucks* and *fingers* and *fudge*, adding a few *fannies* in here and there, willy-nilly, till we'd got all the F-words out of our system.

One cup of tea became two, and then three, as Dottie and I gave Paul all the practical advice we could think of, filling him in on the things that could help, and where he should go, and who it might be good for him to get in touch with.

Paul was exactly like me when I'm interested in something: hungry for all the details, asking all these questions. *What about this? Why does that happen? How do you deal with that . . .*

It could have been knackering – too much, maybe, for most people – but I was hyper-focused, like him, and matching his energy, so I was up for every question he threw at me.

Dottie would join us for a while, then pop out for a fag or a blether with Tommy, leaving us to it – needing a break, I don't doubt, from the two of us and our non-stop jabbering.

Paul had looked me up online, so he seemed to know lots about me already. He'd seen me on *The Late Late Show*, on RTÉ, he said, and he'd watched all the documentaries I'd been in – which was five by now – listing them to me in order of date, telling me which his favourite bits were from each one of them.

'*Fucking stalker!*' I kept ticcing, though it was obvious to me now that Paul wasn't unhinged, just a really nice guy who was desperate for some help.

He was curious to know everything – and I mean every single little thing – about my life, but for some reason it didn't bother me.

I'd got in trouble at times, I said, telling him about the attacks and the fights, how I'd ended up in court and, even though I was acquitted, it was still a horrible thing to have to go through. There was no point pretending.

'What about friends?' he said. 'Do you mind me asking? Do you have any friends? Or does your Tourette's tend to scare them all off?'

'Aye, well, there's that Trotter fella over there, for one,' I said. 'He used to be my boss, didn't you, Tommy?' Tommy waved cheerily back at me, making me tic, '*You fat ginger cunt!*'

'He made the mistake of giving me my job – I've been the caretaker here for years now. It was meant to be temporary, wasn't it, eh, Tommy?' He smiled and rolled his eyes. 'You did nae know what you were letting yourself in for! The fella I was standing in for had an accident and took early retirement, so he ended up getting stuck with me. Anyway, he's no directly responsible for me these days,' I said. 'So, yes, we're mates now. I go over to his, we have a wee barbecue, sit and have a drink in his garden, *talk about his shite boring model buses!*'

'And there's Murray,' Dottie said. 'Dinnae forget Murray.'

'Aye, that's Dottie's son,' I said. 'He's a great pal of mine too, and there's a wee gang of us – we go out, have a drink, play football, that kind of thing.'

'And what about the work you do,' Paul asked, 'with all the Tourette's stuff? Has that helped you, do you think, when it comes to making friends? Has that stopped you from, you know, maybe hiding away?'

'*I hid away from you!*' I ticced. 'Aye,' I said, 'the documentaries have been brilliant for that. I'm not so worried about being out and about in Gala now . . . *out! I'm gay! I'm a gay boy!* You know, because most people have seen them, and now they get what's going on with me. It helps, you know, not to have to keep on explaining yourself, and that's not just me, that's everyone with Tourette's. The more Tourette's is in the public domain . . . *Pubic! Pubic domain!* The more people understand it, the easier life gets for all of us.'

'You should see all the messages he gets,' Dottie said. 'Thousands of them – don't you, John? People with Tourette's from all over the world get in touch with him.'

'*Touch me! Touch my cock!*' I ticced. 'Aye, to share their experiences and say how much the documentaries mean to them.'

'We've been running the weekenders for years now,' I went on, 'and they've really helped to build a community. That's what was missing when I was a kid, a Tourette's community, so it's really massively important to me – *like Dottie, fat slag, you're important to me!* – you know, to keep on building that up.'

I told him about the talks I gave in schools, and for the police – to anyone who'd have me, really – and the work I did as an advisor for Tourette Scotland, which was a big charity these days. There was always something they wanted me to do with them.

'Christ, that's a lot,' Paul said. 'How do you work full-time and find time to do all that?'

'Aye, I had nae realized till I was telling you about it just now,' I said. '*Fucking loads!* Maybe it doesn't feel like a lot – *fucking masses, pal!* Because . . . I dinnae know . . .'

I paused, trying to find the words to sum up in one answer.

'I just love it, pal,' I said, keeping it simple and true.

'I really want to get involved with some of that stuff,' Paul said. 'Do you think there's any way that I can?'

'Aye, well, we've got a weekender coming up here at the community centre,' I said. 'You could always come along to that, see how it all works. I'd be happy to show you the ropes.'

It was dark by the time we left the centre, and I stood for a moment to admire the Christmas lights I'd fixed up around the entrance.

'You've done a lovely job with those lights, Davidson. Best ones ever, I reckon,' Dottie said.

'Cheers, Dottie. Do you know, you're nae wrong about that.'

Walking Paul to his car, I felt a wee twinge of sadness at the thought of saying cheerio to him. I hadn't spent that long, one on one, with another person with Tourette's as full blown as mine in a long time – maybe not ever.

'You're welcome back, Paul, any time. I mean it,' I said as he got into his Vauxhall Vectra.

I really did.

I'd spent years trying to make folk understand what it's like to live with this thing, but Paul didn't need any of that. He already knew. And it hit me, standing there: this was maybe what I'd been missing all along. I'd had people around me who understood for a while, but here was someone who *felt* the same way. It was like seeing myself from the outside. And I knew then, I could just tell, that I'd found a pal for life.

'Cheers, John. I'm going to be taking you up on that – I'd love to see you again,' Paul said with a massive grin, revealing the gap between his two front teeth.

'*That's where you hide your pound coins!*' I ticced, thinking, *That's no what I want to leave him with.*

'Big tits!' he ticced back.

'You've nae neck!'

'Both of you!' Dottie shouted, laughing. 'Enough now – I'm calling time!'

Paul was about to shut his door, when a wee girl walked

past, holding her mother's hand and wearing one of those headbands with reindeer antlers on it.

'Hey!' he shouted, leaning out of his car, so they stopped and stood there, looking at him.

'*Santa's not real, you know!*'

'OK then, Davidson, come on,' Dottie said, linking her arm in mine. 'Time to go.'

37

Birthday

It was a Friday afternoon, and I was just back from work. Usually, I'm done in by the end of the week, and I might have a quick kip on the sofa, maybe zone out for a bit in front of the telly, but not today. Now, I was buzzing, in that restless, 'can't seem to sit still' way that I get when I'm excited about something.

It was the day before my birthday – forty-eight: how did *that* happen? – and I was celebrating up at Dottie's with everyone tomorrow night. *Tomorrow night, though! Ages away! What now?*

I couldn't wait. And I mean, I really *could not* wait. The concept of delayed gratification has always been a mystery to me, so I was brimming with impatience – all tetchy and agitated with it – willing time to fast-forward and just *hurry the fuck up.*

I'd been seeing a fair bit more of my family lately, which was good for all of us, I think. Mum was happier these days, more settled, and it seemed to have made her more generous, because she was taking me out for a pub lunch on Saturday, with Sharon and Caroline too. Even Dad wanted to see me – he'd be popping to mine in the morning, he said – so tomorrow was going to be full-on birthday all the way. *But what about now?*

Tommy! I thought, pacing up and down my sitting room. *I'll call Tommy and get him to come over for a birthday curry with me.*

Why celebrate just the once? Dottie's influence – her mantra about celebrating anything at all, at every opportunity – had clearly rubbed off on me, and I was all over birthdays by now: presents, fancy food, dancing, drinking, the lot. *Bring it all on.*

Come on, I thought, *let's get this party started*, as I called Tommy on his landline, knowing there was no point trying him on his mobile, which, for some frustrating, inexplicable reason, he almost always had turned off.

'Hey, Trotter' – I left a message – 'if you fancy popping down for Indian at mine tonight, give us a call, will you?'

I had my own house now, with a wee garden and no one upstairs or downstairs to be fretting about, so I loved having my mates come round to my place these days.

I tried again, an hour later, leaving another message, probably a bit more urgent-sounding, as I was feeling a wee bit hungry by now. *Come on now, Tommy, get your arse into gear!*

Ach, I bet he's gone to Edinburgh to see his sister, I thought, deflated now, slumping back down on to my couch.

Tommy had slowed down a lot since he'd taken early retirement, his bad leg and diabetes making things increasingly hard for him, but the trips to his sister were the one thing he did regularly. *That's it.*

He'll be in touch tomorrow, I thought, impatient to see the present he'd have bought me. Tommy was always good with gifts – any excuse to indulge his obsession with bargain hunting.

All week he'd been dropping hints to me about trainers. I just hoped I'd got that right, I thought, trying to rub off a mark on the knackered ones I was wearing, eyeing their greying laces. *I could really do with some new trainers.*

I gave him one last try, on his mobile this time, which, as I'd predicted, went straight to answerphone.

The weekend came and went. I had a happy time at Dottie's. Roddy and Murray and Dawn came up, and we had a Chinese and some beers, and there was cake. We all had a right laugh, and I tried to push away the nagging disappointment I felt about Tommy forgetting my birthday – for the first time ever, I realized, since I'd known him.

It disnae matter, I thought, berating myself for being so selfish. *I cannae be mad that he needs a bit of time being looked after by his sister.*

Tommy always put on a good show of being just fine and not needing any help.

'What are you interfering for?' he'd say as I set about cleaning his bathroom or taking out his rubbish. 'Leave it be, will you? I can do it later.' But I'd carry on all the same, and he'd only say it the once because he knew I'd do it anyway, so that was our little ritual we had to go through. He was always grateful when I was done, without directly acknowledging what for, cracking open some beers, asking me to come and join him in the garden, where we'd sit on his wobbly chairs till the sun went down, laughing and blethering about football and cars and all sorts.

Knowing Tommy, he'll call me as soon as he's back, I thought.

Aye, I bet he'll do a belated birthday barbecue for me, something like that.

Knowing Tommy – just thinking those words always gave me a wee flutter of happiness, because I *did* know Tommy, really well, better than most, if I'm honest. Since he'd lost his partner, Ros, a couple of years before, and his mum soon after, apart from his two sisters it was just me, really. I think I was his main person.

I'd worried about Tommy's retirement, fretting about what it could mean for our friendship, but I still saw him all the time. Hard not to, I guess, with his house being right next to the community centre.

Davidson, do you fancy popping in later for a cream cake? He'd call me at work. *I've got myself a couple here*, he'd say. *Ten pence each, they were, from the cooter shelf.*

Tommy was obsessed with that cooter shelf, the place in the supermarket where they put all the food that's just about to go out of date. I was grateful for his obsession, all those after-work cream cakes I enjoyed, and I just loved his proud, smiley face as he presented them to me, asking me to guess – *go on, guess* – the percentage of the discount he'd got on them.

On the Monday morning, I walked past Tommy's house on my way to work and saw his black Škoda Fabia parked outside. *I'll pop by after work*, I told myself, peering at his car, thinking it could do with a clean. *I'll get the Hoover in there later*, I told myself, trying not to let it niggle at me that he hadn't called me as soon as he was home.

Maybe he just stayed longer in Edinburgh, I thought, taking the keys out to unlock the community centre's door. *He's probably only just got back.*

I had Suki by now, another black Lab, as Tilly had sadly passed away the year before. 'Sadly' doesn't even cover it. Losing Tilly knocked the feet from under me. I couldn't go to work for days. When Dottie saw that I wasn't coping, she went and found me a puppy, and took on training her while I was at work. That's what she's like: always, as ever, going above and beyond for me. Like Tilly, Suki was – and still is – my constant companion, always by my side, at work, at home, wherever I went. I just can't imagine my life these days without there being a black Lab in it.

'Shall we go to Tommy's, eh then, Suki?' I said at the end of the day, keys jangling in my pocket as I double-checked, with a twist of the handle, that I'd definitely locked the door. Even now, I could still feel the weight of responsibility when it came to the community centre, finding it hard to believe that I'd been trusted with this, that it was actually me looking after it.

Just the word 'Tommy' had sent Suki nuts with excitement, and now she was barking and weaving in and out of my legs, her tail wagging like crazy.

'Come on then, eh?' I said. 'Let's go see that bastard, shall we?' I followed her as she trotted off down the hill to his house.

Suki knew the drill. She'd sit at Tommy's front door, bark once, and then Tommy would open it, doing his usual 'oh, look who it is' face, before heading off to get her a treat – a massive bone, if she was lucky, or the leftover ham hock he'd have kept from making his Gala-renowned lentil soup.

Suki's first bark didn't do the trick. She looked up expectantly at his door, tail thumping. Then she barked again.

When the door still didn't open, I gave it a knock and

we waited, with Suki whining now, and squirming with excitement.

I knocked again, then tried the handle, and it opened right up.

'Oi! Trotter, are you no speaking?' I called out, sticking my head round the door as Suki pushed past me and ran up the stairs to the sitting room.

'Trotter!' I shouted, following her up the stairs, feeling a bit uncomfortable about being in his house uninvited.

He might be fast asleep on the couch in just his pants, I thought. He was a fiercely private man, so I knew he'd be mad as anything if I found him like that. '*Trotter!*' I called out, louder, just in case.

'Go on then, girl,' I said. *Suki must be feeling awkward too*, I thought, seeing that she'd stopped at the open door to the sitting room and wouldn't go through. 'You can go on in.'

She didn't move. She just stayed there, rigid and alert, and now, as I came up behind her, I could see why.

There was Tommy, lying on the floor, face up, his head against the wall.

All I could think was, *Oh*.

Oh, I thought again, *his carpet needs a good hoover. Oh no, Tommy won't like that.* His burgundy deep-pile carpet was his pride and joy, and rightly so – to be fair, it was beautiful. *He always likes it to look spotless, with the pile all going in the same direction*, I thought. *I'll do that for him in a sec.* I was taking in the way he was lying, with his arms splayed out, in a brand-new white T-shirt – he had an endless supply of new T-shirts – and his trusty grey track-suit bottoms.

There's his Hoover, I thought, seeing it now in the middle of the room. *He shouldn't leave it there – he'll trip over it if he's not careful.*

I don't know how many seconds I stood there, just looking and thinking – well, trying to think, with all appropriate or useful thoughts blocked, because still the only thing I could think, apart from being concerned by the state of his carpet, was, *Oh.*

An indignant bark from Suki jolted me, and then I pushed her out of the way to kneel down beside him.

As soon as I touched Tommy, I knew.

The shock of his cold skin must have switched my frozen brain back on, because now the grief poured into me.

'Oh, Tommy!' I wailed as the sadness came flooding in. 'No, Tommy! No!' I was drowning in it. 'Tommy, don't! You can't – don't do this!'

I tried for a pulse – *just in case, you never know* – and I kept on pressing my fingers against the chill of his wrist, but there was nothing.

Then nothing.

Still nothing.

There was no heart beating in Tommy.

I don't remember what I said when I called 999, only that I did it from his landline, noticing the insistent red flashing light of his answerphone as I spoke.

My messages.

Why didn't I come and check on him sooner? I could have saved him, maybe I could have saved him, I kept thinking. *Why didn't I stop to think that something might have happened?* Hating myself, thinking, *Dottie, I need to call Dottie,* as I stumbled outside to the doorstep, fingers shaking, juddering so hard as I kept on trying to jab at her name on my phone. Missing it, trying again. Missing it.

I was sitting on the doorstep, sobbing, when the ambulance arrived, with Dottie turning up straight after, her face all pink and streaked from crying.

'Oh, John, I'm so sorry.' She scooped me up, hugging me tightly. 'I cannae believe this has happened, can you?' she said as the paramedics rushed inside.

Someone must have called the police, because now here was a police car, screeching to a halt outside. I recognized the policeman walking towards me, checking the buttons on his jacket were done up. It was PC Allan, a tall, blond-haired, serious man who'd been a couple of years above me at school – less tall when I'd last seen him, and a bit blonder, I think, but, even then, always intimidatingly mature and serious.

Maybe it was his uniform, or the reminder of school, perhaps just the massive overriding sadness of it all that set me off, but as soon as I saw him, I felt that familiar pressure building in my throat, and the words forming a sentence. *No, no, no, don't you say it*, I told myself, clamping my mouth shut with one hand, thinking, *Don't talk to me, just don't make me say anything, please.* But he did.

'PC Allan,' he said, straightening up with an officious-sounding cough. 'Is it John Davidson?'

I nodded, biting down hard on my lip as I felt the pressure inside me still building.

'Can you tell me what's happened?' he said, looking past me into Tommy's house.

'I've murdered him!' I shouted. '*He's dead!*'

38

Routemaster

I didn't end up having to grieve for Tommy behind bars, though for a hairy half-hour back there, that was looking like a very real possibility.

Once I'd ticced that I'd murdered Tommy, you should have seen the way PC Allan's eyes lit up. He kind of came alive, and I don't want to say that he was loving it, but *he was clearly fucking loving it* when he announced that the house was now a crime scene and I wasn't to go back inside.

'What do you mean?' I asked, tugging at my hair. *'What do you fucking mean?'*

It wasn't quite right – *unseemly*, Dottie said later – how excited PC Allan was, given that there was Tommy lying dead upstairs. He must have thought that this was his moment, she reckoned. Maybe you'd be hungry for a murder too, she said, if you spent your days picking up drunk Rory Campbell from outside the pub again, and stopping those ne'er-do-well Stewart twins from nicking eyeliners and nail polish from the chemist's.

I remember pacing up and down Tommy's front garden after he said that to me. *'I'm gannae be locked away!'* I shouted as Mrs Wilson from next door walked past. *'It's a crime scene! Watch out, I'm a felon! Get the handcuffs on!'*

I could see PC Allan getting it in the neck – Dottie was tearing strips off him on one side, and the wee female paramedic was on the other, both firing questions at him, proper raging.

'Do you not know about Tourette's?' Dottie was pointing her fingers at him.

'What were you thinking?' the wee paramedic asked. 'Do you no understand what a tic is? Mr Trotter has suffered a heart attack; he's not been murdered,' she said. 'So do you think you owe his poor bereft friend here an apology?'

'In retrospect, I may have been a wee bit hasty back there,' he eventually forced himself to say to me. 'So, yes, Mr Davidson' – he was a bit twitchy and deflated now, after that full-on double assault – 'yes,' he said, clearing his throat, 'you know, I'm sorry about that.'

I had nightmares for weeks after Tommy was gone.

I had to take time off work and move back in with Dottie for a bit, until I could find some way to fully function again.

I dreamt about Tommy every night for a while. The worst of that was that he was alive in my dreams, which were so real, and so vivid, that when I woke up I'd be hit by the loss all over again, so I'd relive it day after day.

The obsessive, OCD part of me kept replaying me finding him, rewinding, playing it back again.

'I should have gone there earlier, Dottie. I could have saved him,' I said, ticcing, 'It's too late now – he's dead! Dead and gone!'

I was torturing myself, Dottie kept telling me.

'You need to let go of this now,' she said. 'You were a great friend to him, John – he said that to me, you know? He said he was lucky to have you.'

Sometimes it can be the very last thing that you want to do that ends up helping you the most. Do you know what I mean?

There was no way in hell that I wanted to go back to Tommy's house again, but his sisters, Mary and Laura, had come down to clear it, and they asked Dottie and me if we'd help them.

I pretended I was fine with it – in as much as I could. 'Aye, Laura, I'd love to,' I said, ticcing, '*No fucking way! Scene of the crime! I'm staying the fuck away!*'

'Oh, I don't want you to come if it's going to upset you, John,' Laura said, her voice full of concern.

'Ach, no,' I said. 'Ignore me, I'm just ticcing, that's all . . . *I'm fucking not! I mean it!*'

We spent a couple of days, the four of us, going through all Tommy's things, and after a while a kind of shift seemed to happen, because the more we talked about him, the lighter things started to feel. The only way I can describe it is that at first it was like Tommy was the elephant in the room, but by the end he just *was* the room, and he was there with us, too, all around us.

Soon we were swapping stories about him, laughing about his obsession with that supermarket cooter shelf, his love of a bargain, howling when we found his massive great stash of identical, unworn T-shirts.

'What are we going to do with all his model buses?' I said, because there were hundreds of the buggers, wherever you looked, displayed in glass cabinets all round his sitting room.

'You can take them if you want,' Laura said.

'*Model buses are for fucking saddos!*' I ticced.

'Do you know, I think I'm with you on that,' she said, laughing.

'I might just have this one, mind,' I said, taking down the Routemaster, turning it over in my hand. 'It reminds me of happy times with him.'

'He's got that photo you took of him behind the wheel of a Routemaster, hasn't he?' Mary said. 'In his bedroom?'

'Aye.' I nodded. 'We had a right laugh on that trip. That was one to remember.'

Tommy had come with me, back in 2007, when I was in the documentary *Tourette de France* – Keith Allen took a group of us with Tourette's round France in an old Route-master. Memorable, aye, though mostly for the wrong reasons. Me and Tommy weren't very happy with how we were portrayed. Still, sometimes it's the mad stuff that sticks in your head.

We had some proper daft moments on that bus.

'I'll call it my birthday present,' I said, slipping it into my jacket pocket. 'He owes me one.'

'I just want to go and do one last thing,' I said, when we were all done and having a final cup of tea in Tommy's kitchen. 'I won't be long.' I took the Hoover out from the cupboard under the stairs, and then headed back up to the sitting room.

I remember the sun was pouring in through his balcony window as I plugged the Hoover in and ran it over that lovely, fluffy burgundy carpet of his, up and down and back again, taking care to make sure it was spotless, with not one speck of dust left on it.

'Just making sure it looks immaculate for you, my old pal,' I said. 'You know, with the pile all going in the same direction. Dinnae worry, OK? I know exactly how it is that you like it.'

39

Back at the Palace

'Dottie.' I was trying to whisper. 'I can't do this.'

I was back in my seat in Holyrood Palace, with my medal, and Dottie was gazing at me with that soppy, watery-eyed look she gives me when she thinks I'm the bee's knees.

'You did it, John, what did I tell you?' Her eyes were still red from crying, and she was dabbing away with a tissue. 'We said, didn't we say you could do it?'

Chris leant across her and patted my shoulder.

'Honestly, we couldn't be prouder of you, John.' His face was all smile; I don't think I'd ever seen his back teeth before.

I wanted to feel all happy and loved up like they were, but I was on edge again, and I couldn't settle for one second.

The Queen hadn't even flinched when I'd shouted out the obscenity, and thank God for that – who'd have thought it? But the whole room was aware of me now – that's what it felt like – and this all-eyes-on-me scenario always gave me this wired, coiled-up, ready-to-pounce feeling, like the clock was ticking and it was just a matter of seconds, a tick and then a tock, before I'd be off again, ticcing too.

There was an elderly lady sitting in front of me, all immaculate in a pale pink suit and matching hat. I kept looking at her, fixating on the back of her head, the string of pearls around her neck, her set white curls poking out from under her hat.

I mustn't punch her, I kept saying to myself, *please God, don't let me hit her*, imagining the scene playing out in slow motion, everyone gasping as I felled her in one blow and she crumpled to the floor. I pictured the rush of people to get to her, and everyone turning, glaring at me, stunned and horrified as I stood up, hands in the air, saying, *Sorry! I didn't mean to, I couldn't help it*, again and again, ripping off my medal then running, as fast as I could, out of the room and away from them all.

I was sitting on both of my hands now. I'd shoved them under my legs and was pressing my thighs down hard on top of them, just in case, though I knew this wasn't a failsafe solution. They'd have had to be tied together for that, with an extra-thick rope just to be sure, with double knots.

'Dottie, *listen to me*.' I could feel the urge building; both my hands were trying to pull out from under me. '*We've got to go!*'

'Yes, of course.' She was standing up already, beckoning to the nearest equerry. She knew that when I said we had to go, that was it, and it was best – often safest – for everyone in the vicinity if she acted quickly, without delay.

'Can I help you, madam?' The equerry leant in.

'It's my son.' I loved it when Dottie called me her son. 'He's too stressed at the minute – he'll hurt somebody if he doesn't get out of here.'

'I understand. Would you please just wait one minute?' he said, before disappearing off through the doors.

'No one's meant to leave before the Queen,' Dottie whispered, nodding towards her, still hard at work handing out the medals.

Moments later the equerry was back again. 'All fine,' he said. 'Please do follow me.'

I bit down hard on my rubber pendant as we made our way past everyone, breathing out a 'Fuck!' of relief as we left the hall and the doors closed behind us.

He led us down the back corridors of the palace until we were outside again and I was squinting in the sunlight as he pushed open the heavy wooden doors.

'Everyone will be joining you here when the ceremony is over,' he said, leaving us at a lovely tree-lined spot outside the chapel.

I looked down at the grass to calm myself – just a minute, to shut out the sensory overload. It was so green and uniform and even; no molehills, no moss, no yellow bits or weeds. It looked like top-of-the-range AstroTurf.

As Dottie and I stood there chatting, I finally started to unwind and take in the full hit of what had just happened, touching the medal again and again, just to check it was real.

'*I've got me a fucking MBE!*' I shouted, as the doors to the palace opened and a stream of people arrived from the ceremony.

Everyone had been invited to have a picnic on the lawns – that was how the day was meant to finish. I really wanted to join them, and it pained me not to be a part of it, but there was no way that could happen. It was hard enough for me to eat at Dottie's, where I mainly still sat in front of the fireplace. The thought of eating in front of people I didn't know, spraying a fancily dressed stranger with a mouthful of mini quiche, made the tics start up in me again.

'*I raped someone!*' I yelled. 'No, I didn't!' I tried not to apologize these days, but always felt the need to add a qualifier after that one.

It was hard not to feel a bit dejected as I watched everyone heading off together to the picnic, but Dottie clocked me, like she always does.

'You haven't forgotten, have you,' she said, putting her arm round me, 'that massive great hamper I've got for us in the boot of the car?'

'It'll taste like *shite*,' I ticced.

'Well, reserve judgement till you've tried one of my vol-au-vents,' she said as we were led to the entrance. 'I reckon they'll give the Queen's a run for their money.'

'*Shite! All shite!*' I yelled, and I went to punch her, but she ducked, and I missed.

'Look at that!' She gave a hoot of laughter. 'I've got ninja skills now, thanks to you! Come on,' she said. 'Let's get to the car and find us a nice place to stop off so we can crack open the champagne.'

As we reached the gate, I clocked a bit of a commotion outside, and straight away I felt myself ease up. It was always a weight off when the drama wasn't mine for once. Two cops were wrestling with a guy who was clearly trying to wriggle free.

Then he looked up, and I just froze. *What the fuck?*

'Oi! John, you fat cunt!'

It was the first time in my life I'd been happy to be called a fat cunt. Paul could have called me anything – he'd come all this way, *just for me*. I couldn't take it in. *I can't believe it.*

'You're all right,' Dottie said to the policemen. 'He's with us. Same condition, same Tourette's as John.'

They looked a bit thrown for a second, then gave a quick nod and let him go.

'I've been waiting for fucking hours!' Paul said, laughing through a riot of jerks and barks and yelps.

'Fucking hours!' I ticced.

'Fuck yeah,' he said, and we ticced back and forth, and it started sinking in as I told him all the details, in between the tics, as we hugged each other and I was crying but trying not to let anyone see, wiping away the hot tears on my sleeve.

'Guess who else has come to see you?' Paul was pointing to a couple of figures coming towards us, and when I saw who they were, the tears started racing down my cheeks too fast for me to even bother to hide them.

Tommy Trotter's sisters, Mary and Laura, had made the journey to see me, too.

'Tommy would have loved this,' Mary said, giving me a teary-eyed kiss.

She looked amazing. They both did. I'd never seen them dressed up like this before.

'Can you imagine how chuffed he'd be for you?' Laura said.

I could picture Tommy's face – his big wide grin – and I knew she was right. He'd have been punching the air for me.

That moment. I still play it over and over in my head, even now.

Here I was, back in the middle, surrounded by people who all knew me for who I was, and who loved me despite that.

The sun was shining down, and I remember I had a bit of a sweat on as I squeezed into the back of Dottie's Volvo, next to Caroline, and wrapped the seatbelt tight around my arm. *No punching.*

I waved goodbye to Paul, who gave me a double thumbs-up

and then flicked me the Vs, and, as the car pulled away, I remember feeling an incredible lightness and realizing it was happiness – that pure and undiluted kind. I felt like I was a ten-year-old kid again, surrounded by my gang of mates, no cares and no worries, flying through the air on my BMX, king of the world.

Epilogue

This story was meant to finish at the end of the previous page, which took us back to me getting my MBE, where we started, tying everything up nicely. *Job done.* But then something happened to me recently which scuppered all that – which almost scuppered everything, and by that I mean me – and I decided it was too important, too unbelievable, in that truth-being-stranger-than-fiction kind of way, to leave out, so here you go . . .

In November 2022, a film director called Kirk Jones contacted me on Facebook. He'd seen my first documentary, *John's Not Mad*, back when he was at school, he said, and it had stuck with him ever since. He was looking for a new project – *What the fuck?* – and he thought my story had the potential to make a great film . . . *Is this for real? Maybe this is some weird kind of convoluted scam?*

He wanted to have a chat with me, he said, and then maybe he could come up and meet me? I had to shut my laptop at that point just to wait for all the explosions to die down in my head.

I was all over the shop – my motor tics in overdrive, whacking the TV, the wall, knocking my mug of tea on to the floor – as I tried to get my head around what had just happened. I kept telling myself, *Hold back, Davidson, calm down. Just speak to the guy first, just fucking wait.*

Kirk seemed like a really genuine guy when we chatted on the phone, and I know I'm good like that – I get a feel for people – but still, I was a wee bit wary. You never know with these film director types, do you? They can be all about the ego, all 'me, me, me', and I had to be careful, mindful of that, because in the wrong hands – with someone who didn't know, or really care, about the reality of my life with Tourette's – I knew it would be way too easy to sensationalize it.

After the call I did a wee bit of humming and hawing with Dottie about it – you know, going through all the what-ifs and stuff, like I do – but in the end, she was like:

'Davidson, just meet the fella, for God's sake. You know what you're like – you'll get a feeling about him either way. What's the worst that can happen? If you've no liked him, you can send him on his way.'

A week later, on Saturday afternoon, Kirk had called me from the airport. He'd said he just needed to pick up the hire car, so he should be with me about two thirty, latest. *Which is now!* I thought, checking the time on my phone for maybe the hundredth time that day. *Which is right this very minute!*

'What's he gannae be like, eh, Suki?' I asked, but Suki was too busy – standing up, then sitting down, then turning round in circles – to even look at me, because she picks up my moods, so she was all restless and keyed up, like I was.

'Fuck me!' I said as I saw this bright neon-pink Fiat 500 turning into the close.

'Suki, that cannae be him,' I said, opening the window and

leaning out to watch as Kirk unfolded himself – all six foot one of him – out of this hilarious wee motor.

'Fucking hairdresser's car!' I ticced, ducking down, thinking, *Shite! Did he hear me or no? Did I maybe get away with it?*

I had another peek out of the window and saw he was outside now, looking up at the houses, trying to work out which one was mine.

'*Wanker!*' I shouted. '*Fucking wanker!*' Well, he knew which one it was now.

I'd opened the door before he could ring the bell, and there he was, this huge, tall, friendly-looking guy with massive hair, all thick and wavy, and big black glasses – you know, the kind that architects and arty people wear.

'I'm Kirk,' he said, as he held out his hand with a big, open smile. 'Nice to meet you.'

'Hi, how are you doing?' I said, shaking his hand. 'Come on in.' I gave myself a wee mental pat on my back, thinking, *Nice one, Davidson, you did well there.*

'Should I take my shoes off?' he said.

'*Let's have sex!*' I ticced, thinking, *Damn, for fucksakes.*

'Should I take my shoes off first?' he said, smiling.

And I leant forward, quick as a flash, and went to punch him in the bollocks, just missing, thank God, though only just.

'I put spunk in there!' I ticced as I handed Kirk his coffee, but by now I'd explained how it's best not to react, so he just gave me a smile and said thank you.

The more Kirk and I chatted, the better I began to feel.

He was kind – you could tell straight away, just by the way he asked questions. Proper thoughtful. And the way he wanted to know everything about Tourette's, how it actually affected me day to day – that really put me at ease.

Dottie called as we were chatting, checking in to see if I was OK.

'Aye, Dottie, you can meet him tomorrow . . . Aye . . . He's going to be taking us all out for lunch, Paul and Murray too.'

I spent the weekend with Kirk and, by the end of it, I just knew. *He felt right.* It was as simple, and as amazing, as that.

Two years later, November 2024, and I'm sitting in a cinema in Galashiels, waiting to watch the rough cut of the film.

'Dottie, I think I need to go,' I said, trying to keep my voice down, because Kirk was sitting right behind us.

'It's OK, John, you'll find it emotional,' she said. 'Of course, it's your life story.'

She didn't understand.

'Just remember those wee clips we've seen,' she said, offering me some popcorn. 'We loved them, didn't we? It's nae gannae be an easy watch for you, but it'll be brilliant, I can feel it.'

That wasn't why I wanted to leave.

'*I'm fucking wabbit!*' I ticced, hoping Kirk didn't know what that meant, as Dottie patted my knee and did the soothing clucky thing she does.

I'd had a chest infection for weeks. I'd been playing it down – no way was I going to delay the screening – but now there was no denying it: I was feeling really, really ill.

I'd been aching all over since I'd woken that morning. I'd tried to ignore it, dosing myself up with paracetamol, but by the time we walked into the cinema I was boiling hot, and my legs felt so heavy, and I could tell from the looks on people's faces that I must be looking really peely-wally with it, too.

I was struggling to breathe as the film started playing, and I was so distracted and panicked by what was going on with me that I couldn't make my mind go still enough to concentrate.

I kept giving it a go, and I focused here and there, ticcing 'I'm an actor!' when I connected with a scene for long enough, and 'You lied to me!' each time a teacher came on screen. There were parts where I got upset and my eyes would fill with tears, but overall I was too ill to take it all in.

By the time the credits rolled, I was worse than ever, and now I was stressing, too, because I knew Kirk would be wanting to have my reaction.

I wanted to be all upbeat and enthusiastic – I could tell, even from the bits I'd taken in, that the film was amazing – but there was nothing, no energy left in me. I couldn't even move my mouth into a smile as I felt Kirk's hand on my shoulder.

'Well?' he said, his face all expectant. 'What do you think?'

'I think that I need to go to hospital,' I said.

I look back at that moment now, and I imagine what that must have done to the poor fella. Of all the reactions he might have gone over in his mind, I dinnae think that would have been on the list.

I can't recall much about leaving the cinema, just Kirk's worried face – fretting about what his film had done to me, I bet – and my legs not working like they were meant to, and how shit scared I was about how hard it was to breathe. I remember asking Dottie, 'What about the after-party?', stressing about missing it, and the guilt because it was me – *it's all my fault* – I'd ruined this massive great big deal of a day.

I was so past caring, I didn't even mind Dottie putting her

arm round me as she guided me to the car. I remember her telling me that she was taking me to the hospital – whispering it, because she knows just how I feel about hospitals. *Everything's going to be OK*, she was saying. *It will all be OK, all right, John? Breathe, keep breathing, we just have to get you there.*

We got to the nearest major hospital just in time.

'Wait there,' Dottie said, dropping me right outside the entrance. 'I'm just going to park the car.'

I was waiting there, like she'd told me to, when I collapsed and had a heart attack.

I had double pneumonia. We didn't know about the heart attack at first, but soon after, a scan revealed a massive blood clot in my heart, and they worked it out backwards from there.

I remember flipping out when I was admitted, shouting, 'I'm not staying! Nobody will understand, no one will get my tics!' and Dottie doing her best to calm me: 'You need to listen to what the doctors are saying, because this is serious, John – you are seriously ill.'

Dottie tried, she really pushed for me to have a private room – my Tourette's was only going to disrupt and upset the other patients, she said – but there was nothing available, so that was it, my worst nightmare: I was going to have to be put on a ward.

Only snatches of that time come back to me. I remember my sister Caroline coming to visit, and my younger brother, William, and Dottie and Chris, but what we talked about, I have no idea. I just remember begging them to get me out, to please find a way to discharge me, too out of it most of the time to understand just how dangerously ill I was.

Sometimes I was more lucid, and at some point I became

aware that there was a man dying in the bed next to me, with all his family gathered round.

I can picture that familiar, panicky sensation I felt, which comes when I'm certain – in this instance, there was no doubt – that I will cause offence.

'You're dying!' I ticced. 'You're gannae die!'

'What did you just fucking say?' the son of the man said, standing up, fists clenched, as he glared at me.

'He cannae help it,' said Dottie, who – thank God – was still with me. 'He's got Tourette's.'

'I ken you've got Tourette's, pal,' the man said, *'but can you no keep your fuckin' mouth shut?'*

Most of that time in the Borders General Hospital has left me; it was too distressing, or I was too ill, maybe both. I think there were times when I understood that I might die – first when they couldn't seem to get the pneumonia in check, and then later when they found out about the state of my heart – though for the most part, I think I was too out of it to care.

Days must have passed – it's hard to know how many – when I came round to see that the dying man wasn't next to me any more, and in his place was another elderly man, who looked a lot like someone I knew.

'I know you! I know that man!' I kept ticcing as I tried to work out how, and who he was, thinking, *That's it, he's a dead ringer for whatshisname, my old teacher, Mr Wainwright*, then ticcing *'Fuck!'* as he turned around and looked my way.

Can it be true? Is this the medication? Am I hallucinating or something? I thought, ticcing *'Fucking bastard!'* as the penny dropped and I realized – *oh my sweet Jesus* – that it *was* Mr Wainwright. My old biology teacher, that prick who'd made my life hell back at school. Here he was, in the bed next to me in hospital, forty-odd years later.

What are the fucking chances of that?

'Ha, ha! Mr Wainwright, you're gannae die!'

He was older and frailer now, but my tics didn't care. 'Karma!' I shouted, remembering the casual cruelty in the way that he'd treated me. 'Karma's a bitch!' I ticced, the humiliation burning away inside me again as I pictured the smirk on his face when he made me stand up on that stool and explain my Tourette's to the whole class, taking the piss the whole time, not stopping the others from piling on too.

'That's it, I'm out!' I said. 'I'm getting the hell away from here!' I ripped off my drip and pushed myself up, took a few shaky steps across the ward, then collapsed.

Once the clot on my heart was discovered, I was blue-lit to the specialist heart hospital in Glasgow, so I could be monitored and given blood thinners to try to stop me from having what they kept calling a 'catastrophic stroke'.

I wished they would stop using that word. *'Catastrophic! I'm catastrophic!'* I kept shouting to myself. *'I'm gannae die soon!'* Because in my own room finally, and in the absence of anyone else to upset, my tics had now turned on me: *'I'll be dead any minute now!'*

I'm back home now, after eight weeks in hospital. It's been a few months, and this whole 'taking it easy' thing has been slow – and I'm not good with slow: *Hurry up, Davidson, you sickly wee bastard!* But I think I'm just about back to myself now.

Soon, I want to sit down with Kirk to watch the film again,

but properly this time, so I can take in every single beautiful second of it. And then I want to watch it all over again, with my family.

But for now, I keep thinking, *I know just how Dottie felt when she made it over the Forth Bridge in one piece . . . I get it. I'm just so grateful and glad to be alive.*

John Davidson, April 2025

Postscript

Back in 2020, a woman called Dr Barbara Morera got in touch with me.

She was conducting a clinical trial with the University of Nottingham, she said. The trial was to test the effectiveness of a wrist-worn device called the Neupulse, which used median nerve stimulation to reduce tics in people with Tourette's syndrome. It had been developed by a spin-out company from the University called Neurotherapeutics Ltd (brand name Neupulse), which had been founded on the work of her Ph.D.

The fifteen-year-old me would have been all *more, more, tell me more*, but I'm more sceptical now, given nothing's worked for me so far; I tend to assume that nothing will.

The device delivers electrical stimulation to the median nerve on the wrist, Barbara explained, which modulates the area of the brain that's altered in individuals with Tourette's syndrome, and this reduces the urge to tic. An initial study with nineteen participants had already shown how effective it was. They were beginning the first trial soon, she said, and she was calling to invite me to take part in it.

I was intrigued. 'Could I have a wee think about it?' I said, wary of jumping straight into something before I knew that much about it.

I read all the literature she sent me, and, as far as I could understand, this device seemed like a much simpler, way less gory/shit-scary option than deep brain stimulation, an invasive operation involving a hole being drilled in your skull and having areas of your brain stimulated while you're conscious. I'd actually been considering this at one point, which gives you an idea of how desperate I've been, because I'm dead squeamish when it comes to operations and stuff, and the thought of my brain being opened up while I'm awake is the stuff of nightmares to me. But if your real life is the stuff of nightmares sometimes, then it's surprising the things you'll consider . . .

I said yes, I'd love to take part in the trial.

The feeling was instant.

Wow. Oh my God. This is amazing! Those were my first thoughts when I put the band on.

Everything felt . . . just right.

The world felt different.

My mind quietened down.

I stopped scanning my environment.

I could think clearly.

I started laughing, then giggling like a wee kid.

'What is it?' Barbara said.

'You have no idea.' My cheeks were aching, I was grinning that hard. 'Oh man, honestly, this feels amazing.'

And I was so carried away with just how amazing it felt, I didn't even notice that ten minutes had passed and I hadn't ticced, not even once.

I took part in a couple of different studies which took eight weeks in total. I wore a device that looks a bit like a Fitbit, which I strapped to my wrist for fifteen minutes a day for the first trial, and in the second, I could wear it for as long as I wanted. It's a flexible device, designed to be used as little or as much as is needed, which I liked, as, once I'd got used to it, I only felt the need to wear it when I was going anywhere public.

I still ticced from time to time, but the tics were nothing like as aggressive and loud as they used to be. Without the band, I shouted 'Fuck!' Now, I just said it under my breath, so my tics completely lost their shock value.

My compulsions were gone, too. Well, not exactly gone; I still had the same thoughts – about knocking a glass off the side, testing a blade, whacking someone in the face, that kind of thing – but now I'd lost the desire to act on them.

I could go out now and not have to worry about offending anyone, or drawing any unwanted attention.

In the nicest possible way, I disappeared.

I cried when I had to give the band back.

I'm not good at waiting – I'm still *really fucking bad* at waiting – and the band's not being released until 2026.* But I'm telling you, when it's out, I'll be first in the queue.

I'm cautious about getting my hopes up these days, but trust me: it's going to be life-changing.

---

* More information about the band can be found at www.neupulse.co. Results of the clinical trial that John took part in showed not only an immediate reduction of symptoms from participants while receiving stimulation but also a reduction of symptoms after four weeks of using the device for ten minutes a day. This showed immediate and sustained benefits from the stimulation.

   The clinical trial included 135 participants, and the results showed a reduction of average 25 per cent in tic frequency while receiving stimulation (immediate benefit) and a reduction of average 35 per cent in tic severity after four weeks of ten minutes of daily stimulation (sustained benefit).

   The expected release date is early 2026 in the UK, with the US and Europe to follow, after the appropriate regulatory approvals.

Acknowledgements

I'd like to give my heartfelt thanks to my parents for giving me life.

To Dottie, Chris, Dawn, Murray and Roddy – thank you for taking me in and making me part of your family. You saved me from a very shaky period in my life and I love you all so much.

To my late best pal, Tommy Trotter – I miss you every day, big man. You were my go-to for advice, for a shoulder to cry on, and for just laughing at life's madness.

Rest in peace, Stu (Chopper). And rest easy, Sparky boy.

To Mary and Laura, Tommy's sisters – thank you for all your support over the years. The visits you made to Galashiels even after Tommy passed, and the stories you shared about growing up with him, meant the world to me.

To everyone at Langlee Community Centre, where I've worked for the past thirty-four years – thank you. And to all the committee members – thanks for trusting me to look after this incredible building at the heart of our community.

A special thank-you to Dr Ramaj, who is sadly no longer with us. You were the matriarch of our community for so many years. I learned so much from you, and you're sorely missed.

To my brilliant next-door neighbours, Pauline and Jan – thanks for putting up with my impulsivity, my wild stories, and for patiently explaining everything involving tools and heavy lifting.

A big thank-you to Kate Hordern at KHLA, and to Dr Barbara Morera, Ph.D. at Neurotherapeutics Ltd.

Working on this book has been an unforgettable experience. Thank you to everyone at Transworld Publishers who has been involved with it. I'm so glad I chose Transworld: as soon as I met Susanna Wadeson I felt that I could trust her implicitly to do a great job, and I'm happy to say I was right! Thanks to the editorial team: Kate Samano, Eleanor Updegraff, Katherine Cowdrey, Holly Reed and Dan Balado. Thanks to Phil Lord for the inside page design, Cat Hillerton in production, James Jones and Marianne Issa El-Khoury for the jacket design. Thanks to Patsy Irwin for the publicity, to Hannah Winter and Ross Ainsworth in marketing and Tom McWhirter for the audio. You have all played a vital part in the making of a book that I'm incredibly proud of.

I want to give special thanks to the writer Abbie Ross, who worked on the book with me. Abbie's not just a writer but a psychotherapist too, and from the very start her warmth, empathy and understanding put me completely at ease. I knew the moment we met that we'd work well together – and as the weeks went by, I found myself opening up about things I've never talked about before. She just got it. The more we worked, the less I had to explain. She seemed to instinctively understand what living with Tourette's is like.

Working with Abbie has been both therapeutic and full of laughs – she's the best listener and has the most brilliant sense of humour, which meant I never had to second-guess myself or worry about how I came across. Her deep understanding of ADHD meant I felt understood in a way I hadn't expected.

It's been remarkably easy and genuinely enjoyable, and I feel lucky to have had her alongside me in telling this story. I have Kirk Jones, the director of the film *I Swear*, to thank for recommending her – and I'll be forever grateful to him, because I honestly can't imagine a better person to have worked with.

Thank you.

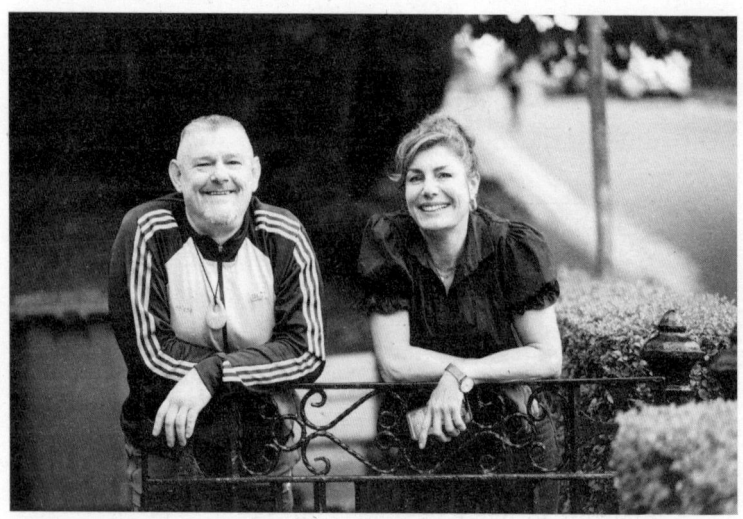

I SWEAR

NOW A MAJOR NEW FILM

A KIRK JONES FILM

STARRING:
ROBERT ARAMAYO
MAXINE PEAKE
WITH SHIRLEY HENDERSON
AND PETER MULLAN

Kirk Jones' emotionally engaging, funny and compelling new film I Swear charts John Davidson's Tourette's diagnosis at the age of 15 years old. Beginning with the onset of John's condition in the early 1980s, the film follows him through his troubled teens and early adulthood, and explores this little known and entirely misunderstood condition, along with his attempts to live a 'normal' life against the odds.

COMING SOON TO CINEMAS

ONE STORY HIGH   TEMPO   STUDIOCANAL
A CANAL+ COMPANY

John Davidson MBE was born in 1971 in Galashiels. After leaving school without qualifications, he began work as a caretaker at Langlee Community Centre in Galashiels, where since 2002 he has also been a part-time youth worker.

Aged sixteen, John was the subject of a BBC documentary, *John's Not Mad*, about living with Tourette's syndrome, and he has since been an ambassador for the condition, giving talks and workshops in schools and to the police, and running residential camps for young people with Tourette's. Since 1989 he has featured in several follow-up documentaries; Kirk Jones's 2025 film *I Swear* is based on John's life.

In 2019 John joined the board of Tourette Scotland and was awarded an MBE in recognition of 'his efforts to increase understanding of the condition and helping families deal with it across the country'. He has also gained international recognition for his online support for families all over the world.